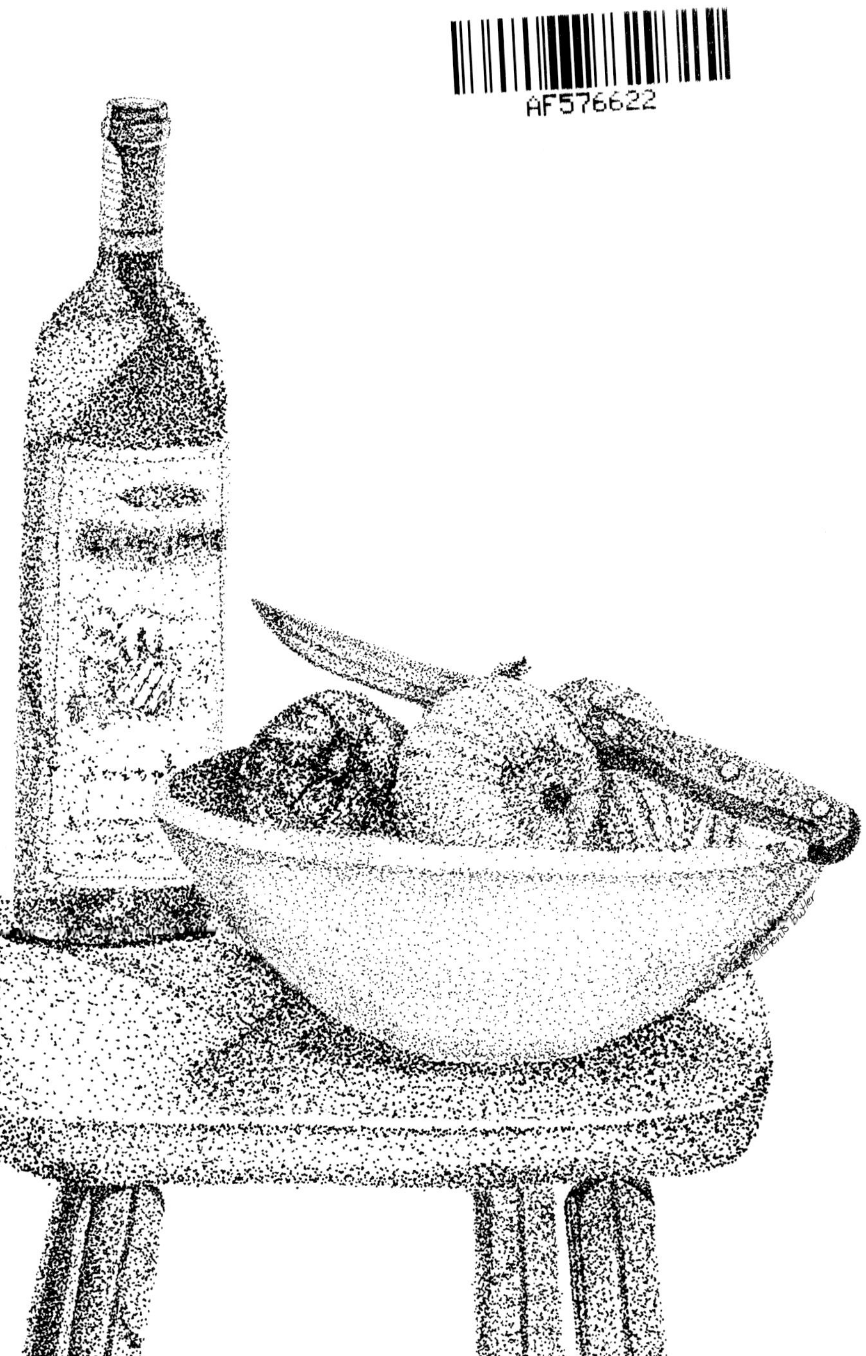

The Power of Prevention Cookbook

We have taken the pains to find out such a multitude of different foods which were unknown to our ancestors that we have introduced a cloud of diseases which they knew nothing of.

Dr. M. L. Lemery

A Treatise of All Sorts of Foods, 1745

The Power of Prevention Cookbook

A Return to Traditional Healthy Eating for the 21st Century

Sandra J. Dickerson

Illustrated by Amanda Clements Butler

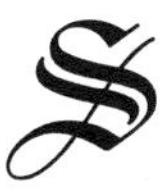

Saville Books

Georgetown, Washington, D.C.

First Printing June 1991

Printed in the United States of America

Library of Congress Cataloging in Publication Data

Dickerson, Sandra J. (Sandra Jean), 1964- *The Power of Prevention Cookbook: a return to traditional healthy eating for the 21st century*/Sandra J. Dickerson; illustrations by Amanda Clements Butler; with an introduction by Oliver Alabaster, M.D.

p. cm. Includes Index

1. Low-fat diet—Recipes. 2. High-Fiber diet—Recipes. I. Title
RM237.7.D53 1991 90-19500
ISBN 0-929693-02-7 $22.00 (H)
ISBN-0929693-03-5 $15 (PBK)
641.5'63—dc20 CIP

Library of Congress Catalog Card Number 90-19500
International Standard Book Number 0-929693-02-7 (HC)
International Standard Book Number 0-929693-03-5 (PBK)

Saville Books

Two Thousand South Second Street
Arlington, Virginia 22204-1959
(703) 271-8778

P.O. Box 25403
Georgetown, Washington, D.C. 20007

For my husband, Robert who has taught me the value and necessity of responsible eating.

Acknowledgments

The Cancer Research Foundation of America and specifically Carolyn Aldigé have been the cornerstone of this project. Without the financial and professional support offered through the CRFA, this cookbook would not have been possible. I am truly appreciative of the role the administration of the foundation has played in bringing these recipes to the public.

I extend my heartfelt appreciation to Oliver Alabaster, M.D. for his expertise, support and encouragement from the outset of this book.

I am quite grateful to Michael B. Albert, M.D. for his assistance over the last few years and for his enthusiasm for the message of healthy eating.

For her artistic talent and graphic contributions, I extend my special thanks to Amanda Clements Butler.

Thank you to my wonderful long-standing friends, Gerald M. Zamborowski, Esq., Deborah A. Milbreath and Loretta Zamborowski, who have provided emotional support and encouragement for many years and especially during the creation of this book.

My sincere thanks to John M. DiJoseph, Esq., and Patricia M. Drost, Esq., for their friendship and professional services which have meant so much.

Finally, I would like to thank my mother-in-law, Anna J. Dickerson, for her love which will always be a great strength to me.

Acknowledgments

Introduction

There is now abundant evidence that what we eat makes an enormous difference to our risk of developing premature illness such as heart disease and cancer. In *The Power of Prevention Cookbook* you will discover a wonderful selection of recipes that incorporate everything we know about how to use food to maintain optimum health and vitality -- just as our ancestors used to do!

If we look at medical progress over the past 100 years, it is clear that the common diseases such as cancer and heart disease that afflict so many of us today were rare in the past. In fact, 100 years ago half the population was dead before the age of 40 mainly due to infectious diseases, not heart disease or cancer; now that number is down to 3%!

You might think that this dramatic medical progress in terms of increased life expectancy was due to advances in treatment, but the real reasons were almost entirely due to preventive health measures such as better sanitation, better living conditions and vaccination programs. Despite this impressive evidence that prevention is the most important aspect of healthcare for the American population, only 0.3% of the present healthcare budget of $600 billion goes toward prevention; the rest is spent extravagantly on the most costly healthcare system in the world.

This costly approach to healthcare makes even less sense when we realize that 80% of deaths before the age of 75 are due to cancer and heart disease, and that we have the power to reduce these deaths by nearly 70% through prevention!

Where, who or what is the culprit? Well, tobacco and bad dietary habits are equally responsible for this premature illness; and we certainly have the power to do something about this. Instead, many people look to industrial pollution or hereditary factors as being responsible because it is easier to blame something over which we have no control and no responsibility.

This has now changed. Starting with *The Power of Prevention*, which is also published by Saville Books, I described how important it is to change the balance of the American diet to reduce the risk of cancer and heart disease. This simple book provides the reader with a good understanding of the importance of dramatically reducing dietary fat, increasing dietary fiber, and increasing the intake of fruits, vegetables, and whole grain or bran cereals. Of all these changes, reducing fat is the hardest to do, because fat is everywhere in the American diet. Even knowledgeable nutritionists usually don't count the fat accurately, especially when they are eating out or following recipes. How then can we expect the public to follow recommendations to reduce their fat intake?

The answer is of course *The Power of Prevention Cookbook!* Here you will find recipes that take the thinking out of healthy eating. You will do wonders for your health and your enjoyment of good food by using these low fat, high fiber recipes. Each recipe is also accompanied by a detailed nutritional analysis for those readers who want to count the grams of fat or fiber as well as the vital vitamins that they consume each day, all of which may contribute significantly to influencing the risk of disease in the future.

Details of just how much protein, fat, fiber and vitamins you need each day are found in the accompanying volume *The Power of Prevention,* but you should aim to limit your fat intake to about 50 grams per day (don't forget to check the food labels when you shop); and you should increase your fiber intake to the recommended level of about 25-35 grams per day.

Finally, a unique feature of this cookbook is the presence of recipes that use Alpine Lace® FREE N' LEAN™ non-fat cheeses. These delicious cheeses allow you to get the calcium you need without the harmful fat. Now you will be able to entertain your family and your friends with the healthiest recipes to be found anywhere.

Oliver Alabaster, M.D.

Director, The Institute for Disease Prevention

Washington, DC

Foreward

Since the publication of Dr. Oliver Alabaster's *The Power of Prevention*, there has been a substantial number of published reports which show that not only is a diet that is high in fat detrimental to health, but that the level which was previously thought to be acceptable, might in fact be dangerously high for many people!

When Dr. Alabaster cited the report, *Dietary Goals of the United States*, which recommended a dietary fat level of 30%, he was prophetic when he correctly asked ". . . just what [are] the government nutritionists afraid of?" The answer to his far reaching question may lie in the fact that until now, most people equated low-fat diets with a lack of taste, deprivation and recipes which rely on foreign and often unfamiliar ingredients.

Furthermore, Sandra J. Dickerson observed that while it is possible to lower the intake of fat to one half of that 30% recommendation, and even lower, those who do, often have a low rate of compliance and gradually return to a regimen that includes those fatty ingredients which are more familiar to them such as meat and whole-milk dairy and cheese products.

When in late 1990 reports began to surface of additional health benefits that can be derived from diets which are very low in fat (fewer than 10% of the calories), Dickerson began to supplement and improve her recipes to make them both familiar to the average person, and great tasting!

No longer does the person who wants to drastically cut his intake of fat have to rely on such ubiquitous fare as brown rice as the main course, seaweeds [the macrobiotic fringe], tofu and tempeh as the mainstay for every recipe.

In fact, *The Power of Prevention Cookbook* includes such a vast array of familiar and favorite recipes that it can and should be used for the entire family as well as for entertaining guests. With the introduction of a non-fat cheese to the market in 1990 - Alpine Lace® FREE N'LEAN™ by First World Cheese, Inc., Dickerson not only recommends cheese, she makes it a cornerstone of a new way of life which is sure to reap health benefits for all who choose to follow it.

The Power of Prevention Cookbook is the first low-fat cookbook to include recipes which were previously shunned by those wanting to improve health or reduce their risk of heart attack, stroke, cancer, premature aging and a host of other health problems. Consider just a few of the more than 200 entries: **Blue Cheese Spread**, **Fettuccine**, **Spaghetti Carbonara**, **Cheese Pizza**, **Lasagna**, **Cheese Sauce for vegetables**, and such desserts as **Turnovers**, **Cakes**, **Cobbler**, and even the almost always forbidden **Cheesecake** made with real cheese!

The Power of Prevention Cookbook will not only become a cornerstone of your new way of eating -- which will contribute enormously to your present and future overall health, but will also help you to demonstrate to your family and friends that a healthy diet need not be one of abstinence and deprivation. Perhaps it will also inspire them to join you in a more healthy way of eating!

About The Author

Sandra J. Dickerson lives in Washington, DC where she works for an association management firm on an allied health related account. She is currently completing a screenplay and a series of children's books.

Note to the Cook

Remember, one good way to reduce the amount of fat in your diet is to use non-stick vegetable spray instead of oil. If oil is not recommended in the recipe, use vegetable spray on all cooking surfaces. You may want to try vegetable spray in place of oil in some of your favorite dishes.

Also, try cutting the amount of oil, butter or margarine in half (or less) when preparing recipes from other cookbooks. You'll be surprised at how little change there is in taste and what a difference there is in the percentage of calories derived from fat.

Why not try a new make-over for an old dish? Add carrots or spinach to whatever dish you are preparing whenever possible. They will add new color, good taste and improved nutritional benefits.

I hope you enjoy these recipes and find them not only great tasting, but beneficial to your health.

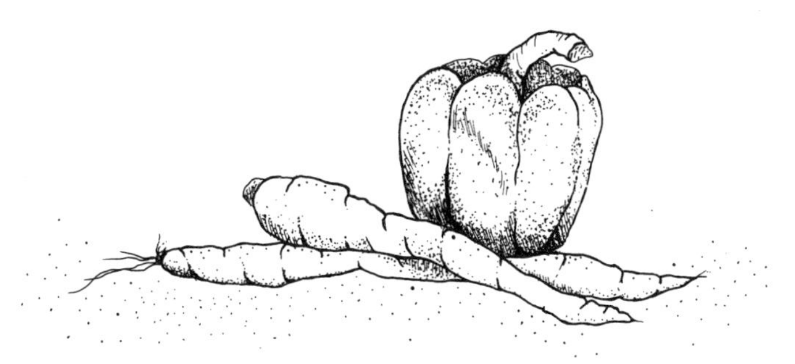

Table of Contents

The Main Course

FREE N'LEAN Cheese

Appetizers and Hors D'oeuvres

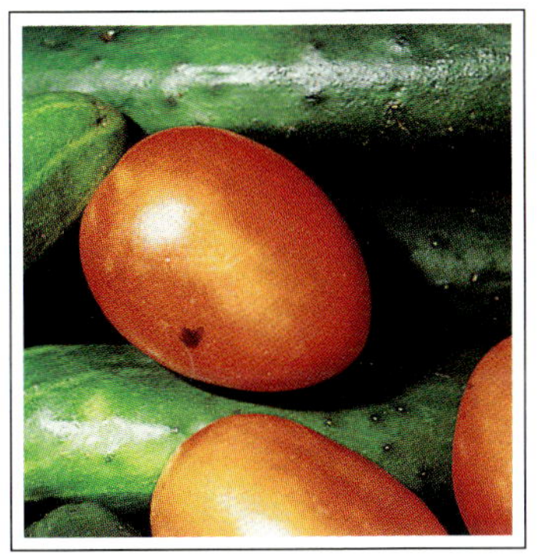
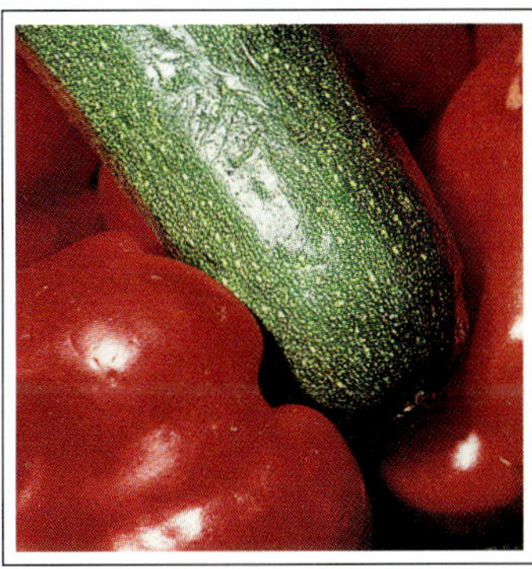
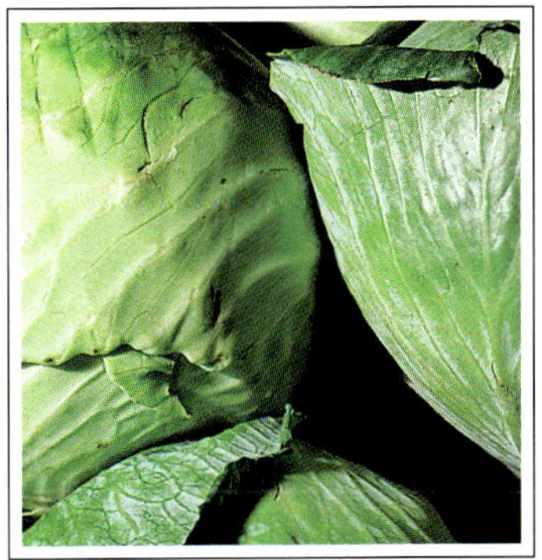
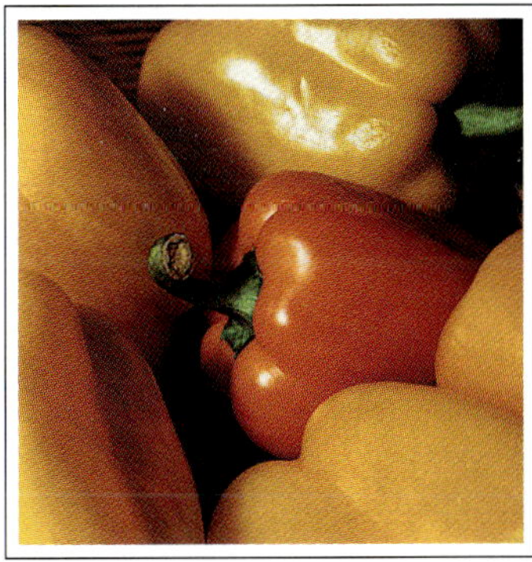

Bean Dip

3 cups Pinto Beans

1 pressed clove of Garlic

4 tablespoons Salsa Sauce

Soak beans overnight in refrigerator. Cook for 2 hours and 45 minutes at a gentle boil. Drain into colander. Cool to room temperature. Place in food processor. Using the steel blade attachment, process until beans are a thick, spread-like consistency. Add garlic and salsa sauce. Blend again. Place in bowl. Garnish with a sprig of mint.

Number of Servings: 4
Nutritional Analysis Per Serving:
Calories: 162
Fat: trace
Fiber: 13 gm
Cholesterol: -0-
Saturated Fat: -0-
Beta Carotene: 150 I.U.
Vitamin C: -0-

Blue Cheese Spread

1 7.5 oz. package of Non-Fat Farmer's Cheese

1 oz. Blue Cheese

1 shredded Carrot

Using softened farmer's cheese, blend in blue cheese until mixture is very smooth and creamy. Add shredded carrot and mix until it is dispersed throughout the cheese for color and nutritional benefits.

Number of Servings: 4
Nutritional Analysis Per Serving:
Calories: 65
Fat: 2 gm (31%)
Fiber: 1 gm
Cholesterol: 8 mg
Saturated Fat: 1 gm
Beta Carotene: 5,100 I.U.
Vitamin C: 3 mg

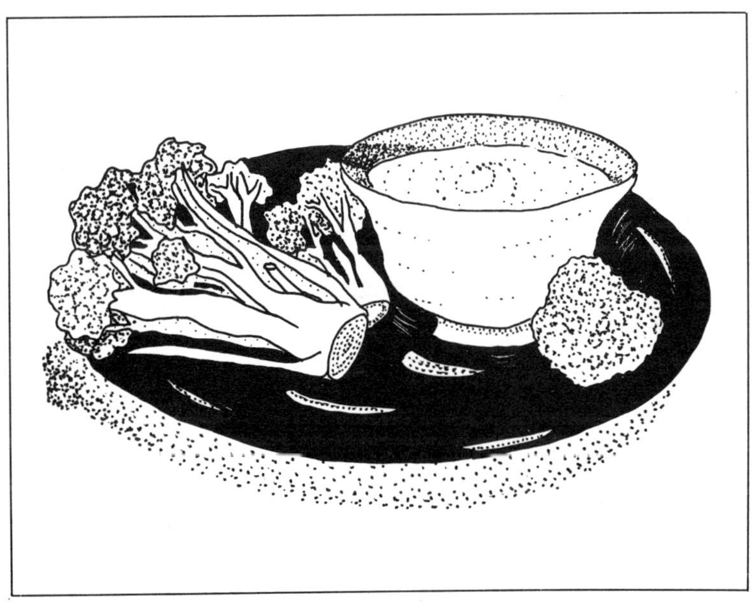

Winter Broccoli Dip

Winter Broccoli Dip

1 head of Broccoli

1 cup Beef Bouillon

1 cup drained Non-Fat Yogurt

Dash of Tabasco Sauce

Place broccoli flowerets in generous amount of water and boil for 10 minutes. Drain, reserving 1/2 cup broccoli broth. Dissolve bouillon cube in broth. In blender combine broccoli, broth and yogurt. Blend until mixture is smooth. From time to time, stop the blender and, using a spatula, scrape the sides of the container so that mixture is completely blended. When finished, pour into saucepan and stir in a dash of Tabasco Sauce. Warm to serving temperature. Pour into fondue pot. Serve with Vegetable Bouquet.

Number of Servings: 2
Nutritional Analysis Per Serving:
Calories: 170
Fat: 1.5 gm (8%)
Fiber: 3 gm
Cholesterol: 1 mg
Saturated Fat: -0-
Beta Carotene: 3,000 I.U.
Vitamin C: 100 mg

Creamy Dilled Cucumbers

1 thinly sliced Cucumber

1 8 oz. container Non-Fat Yogurt

1/4 teaspoon Dillweed

Mix non-fat yogurt and dillweed. Stir all ingredients together and let marinate overnight in a sealed container.

Number of Servings: 2
Nutritional Analysis Per Serving:
Calories: 92
Fat: -0-
Fiber: 1 gm
Cholesterol: 1 mg
Saturated Fat: -0-
Beta Carotene: 35 I.U.
Vitamin C: 4 mg

Cucumber Dip

2 peeled, chopped Cucumbers

1 8 oz. container Non-Fat Yogurt

1/4 teaspoon Dillweed

Dash of Garlic Salt

Dash of Onion Salt

In a food processor, using steel blade, mash cucumbers. When cucumbers have reached a liquid, but lumpy stage remove from food processor. Add remaining ingredients and stir until well mixed. Serve with carrot and celery stalks.

Number of Servings: 4
Nutritional Analysis Per Serving:
Calories: 50
Fat: -0-
Fiber: 1 gm
Cholesterol: 2 mg
Saturated Fat: -0-
Beta Carotene: 60 I.U.
Vitamin C: 3 mg

Spanish Endive

6 Endive

2 tablespoons of Blue Cheese

2 tablespoons Non-Fat Farmer's Cheese

1 tablespoon Red Wine Vinegar

In a small bowl combine 1 tablespoon each of blue cheese and farmer's cheese. Add small amount of red wine vinegar. Begin to stir the three ingredients together. When mixture begins to look smooth and liquid, add the remaining tablespoon of blue cheese and farmer's cheese. Stir. Add the remaining portion of red wine vinegar. Stir until mixture is very smooth. Pour cheese sauce into a small clear bowl with high sides. Separate endive leaves. Beginning on the outside, line bowl with the largest endive leaves. Working in a circle, toward the center, add endive leaves until center is full (put the smaller leaves in the center). This is a lovely dish for the table because it looks like a flower and is quite easy to manage since cheese and endive are in one bowl.

Number of Servings: 4
Nutritional Analysis Per Serving:
Calories: 43
Fat: 2 gm (41%)
Fiber: .5 gm
Cholesterol: 6 mg
Saturated Fat: 1 gm
Beta Carotene: 1,100 I.U.
Vitamin C: 5 mg

Eggplant Dip

8 cups diced, peeled Eggplant

1 coarsely chopped Green Pepper

2 stalks of Celery, chopped

1 chopped Onion

1 8 oz. can of Tomato Sauce

1/4 cup Water

2 teaspoons Sugar

Using non-stick spray sauté onion in skillet until tender. Add tomato sauce, water and sugar. When mixture starts to bubble slightly add eggplant, green pepper and celery. Allow to simmer on low temperature for 20 - 30 minutes. Chill before serving.

Number of Servings: 4
Nutritional Analysis Per Serving:
Calories: 100
Fat: trace
Fiber: 3 gm
Cholesterol: -0-
Saturated Fat: -0-
Beta Carotene: 840 I.U.
Vitamin C: 39 mg

Herb and Cheese Spread

1 7.5 oz. package of Farmer's Cheese

1 teaspoon of Thyme

1 teaspoon of Rosemary

1 teaspoon Black Pepper

1 tablespoon Olive Oil

In a large bowl combine farmer's cheese (at room temperature), herbs, pepper and olive oil. Stir until well mixed. Place in air tight container and marinate overnight. Do not store longer than two weeks.

Number of Servings: 4
Nutritional Analysis Per Serving:
Calories: 60
Fat: 3 gm (45%)
Fiber: -0-
Cholesterol: 2 mg
Saturated Fat: less than 1 gm
Beta Carotene: 100 I.U.
Vitamin C: -0-

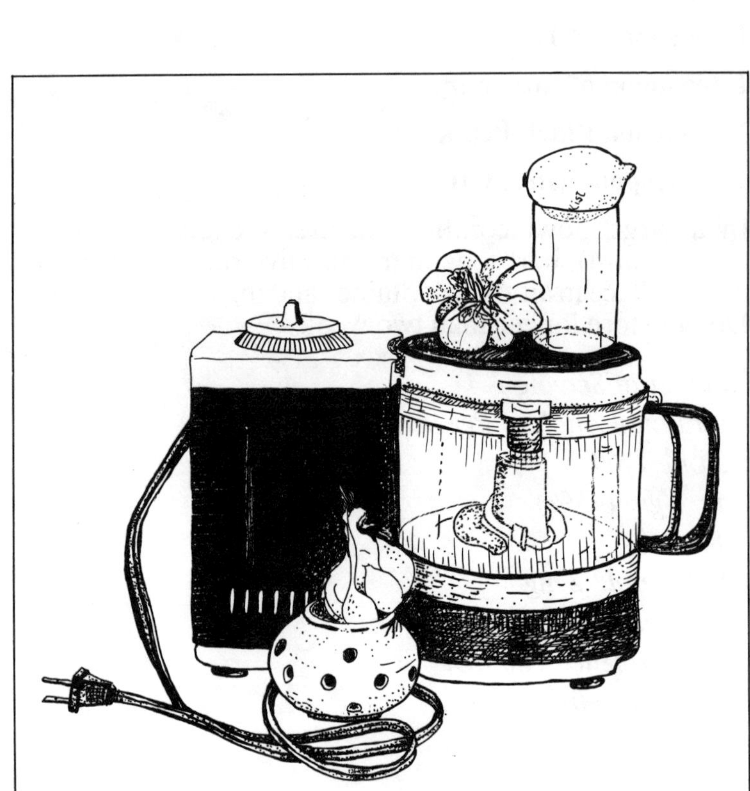

Hummus

Hummus

1 15 oz. can of Garbanzo Beans

1 pressed clove of Garlic

4 tablespoons Tahini

Drain and rinse beans in colander. Place in food processor. Using the steel blade attachment, process until beans are a thick, spread-like consistency. Add garlic and tahini. Blend again. Place in bowl. Garnish with a sprig of parsley.

Number of Servings: 4
Nutritional Analysis Per Serving:
Calories: 225
Fat: 10 gm (10%)
Fiber: 6 gm
Cholesterol: -0-
Saturated Fat: 1 gm
Beta Carotene: 10 I.U.
Vitamin C: -0-

Moje

2 Italian Tomatoes (grated without skin)

1/2 finely chopped Purple Onion

2 pressed cloves of Garlic

2 teaspoons Red Vinegar

1 tablespoon Olive Oil

Dash of Salt

In large bowl, combine all ingredients. Serve with warm bread.

Number of Servings: 2
Nutritional Analysis Per Serving:
Calories: 98
Fat: 7 gm (64%)
Fiber: 1 gm
Cholesterol: -0-
Saturated Fat: less than 1 gm
Beta Carotene: 695 I.U.
Vitamin C: 26 mg

Smooth Onion Dip

1 cup Farmer's Cheese or Plain Low-Fat Cottage Cheese

1/2 cup chopped Onion

3 tablespoons Skim Milk

Dash of Cayenne Pepper

Place all ingredients listed above in food processor. Process until smooth. Place in small bowl or crock, garnish with fresh herb sprig. Best if allowed to marinate overnight in refrigerator in air-tight container.

Number of Servings: 2
Nutritional Analysis Per Serving:
Calories: 85
Fat: less than 1 gm (5%)
Fiber: less than 1 gm
Cholesterol: 5 mg
Saturated Fat: less than 1 gm
Beta Carotene: 65 I.U.
Vitamin C: 4 mg

Sesame Seed Spinach

2 pounds of Spinach

1 tablespoon Toasted Sesame Seeds

1 tablespoon Sesame Oil

2 tablespoons Soy Sauce

1 bunch of Scallions, chopped

Place spinach in small amount of water. Allow to cook until wilted. Drain in colander until cool. In a large bowl combine spinach, sesame oil and soy sauce. Mix thoroughly. Place in serving dish. Top with scallions. Sprinkle with sesame seeds.

Number of Servings: 6
Nutritional Analysis Per Serving:
Calories: 62
Fat: 4 gm (52%)
Fiber: 3 gm
Cholesterol: -0-
Saturated Fat: less than 1 gm
Beta Carotene: 13,000 I.U.
Vitamin C: 11 mg

Shredded Carrot Spread

1 cup Low-Fat Cottage Cheese

6 grated Carrots

2 tablespoons Skim Milk

Dash of Parsley Flakes

Shred carrots as finely as possible. Using the same bowl the carrots were shredded in, combine carrots, cottage cheese and skim milk very well. Place in serving dish. Sprinkle very lightly with parsley flakes.

Number of Servings: 4
Nutritional Analysis Per Serving:
Calories: 80
Fat: less than 1 gm (3%)
Fiber: 1 gm
Cholesterol: 2 mg
Saturated Fat: less than 1 gm
Beta Carotene: 30,000 I.U.
Vitamin C: 11 mg

Tofu Sandwich Spread

1 pound package of Soft Curd Tofu

2 boiled Eggs (use whites only)

2 tablespoons Reduced-Fat Mayonnaise

2 shredded Carrots

1 stalk of Celery, chopped

1/4 teaspoon Ground Black Pepper

Dash of Soy Sauce

In large bowl, using fork, break apart block of tofu. Remove yolk from boiled eggs (boil eggs for five minutes), thinly slice egg whites, add to tofu. Add remaining ingredients. Stir until well combined.

Number of Servings: 10
Nutritional Analysis Per Serving:
Calories: 48
Fat: 3 gm (48%)
Fiber: .5 gm
Cholesterol: -0-
Saturated Fat: less than 1 gm
Beta Carotene: 4,000 I.U.
Vitamin C: 2 mg

Tzaziki

1 8 oz. container of Plain Non-Fat Yogurt

1 peeled, chopped Cucumber

2 pressed cloves of Garlic

Strain yogurt through cheesecloth for approximately six hours in refrigerator. Mix together cucumber and garlic; combine with strained yogurt. Discard left-over water from yogurt. Best if marinated overnight. Store in air-tight container, not longer than one week.

Number of Servings: 4
Nutritional Analysis Per Serving:
Calories: 35
Fat: trace
Fiber: less than 1 gm
Cholesterol: 1 mg
Saturated Fat: less than 1 gm
Beta Carotene: 10 I.U.
Vitamin C: 2 mg

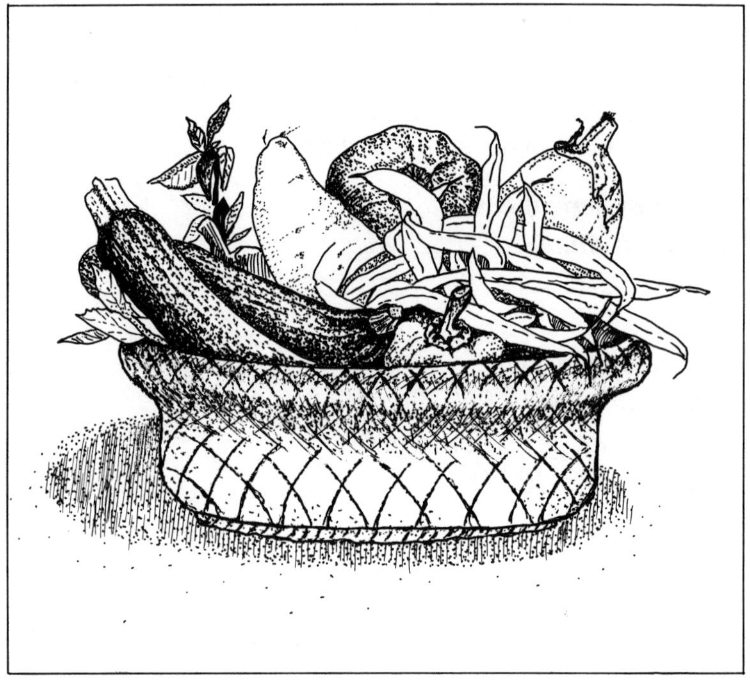

Vegetable Bouquet

Vegetable Bouquet

1 head Broccoli

1 head Cauliflower

8 Carrots

2 bunches of Celery

1 pound Green Beans

3 bunches of Scallions

Prepare vegetables as follows:

* Clean and cut broccoli and cauliflower into flowerets
* Clean and peel carrots, cut into thin strips
* Clean and cut celery into 3 inch sections
* Clean and cut the ends off green beans
* Clean and cut roots off scallions

Number of Servings: 12
Nutritional Analysis Per Serving:
Calories: 30
Fat: less than 1 gm (9%)
Fiber: 2 gm
Cholesterol: -0-
Saturated Fat: less than 1 gm
Beta Carotene: 16,000 I.U.
Vitamin C: 41 mg

Vegetable Pâté

2 cups finely grated Carrots

1 cup finely chopped Celery

1 cup finely minced Onion

3 cups cooked, drained Garbanzo Beans

3 pressed cloves of Garlic

4 chopped Scallions

3 tablespoons Olive Oil

1/2 cup Bread Crumbs

1/2 cup Plain Non-Fat Yogurt

3 tablespoons Parsley

1 teaspoon Thyme

Preheat oven to 325 degrees. Using non-stick spray sauté carrots, celery, onion and garlic over medium heat until soft. Place garbanzo beans and scallions in food processor, process until smooth using steel blade attachment. Combine all ingredients in large bowl, mix well. Place contents of bowl in loaf pan sprayed with non-stick spray, cover with foil and bake for 45 minutes. Allow pan to cool before removing paté. Pâté may be served warm or chilled.

Number of Servings: 20
Nutritional Analysis Per Serving:
Calories: 75
Fat: 3 gm (30%)
Fiber: 2 gm
Cholesterol: less than 1 mg
Saturated Fat: less than 1 gm
Beta Carotene: 3,175 I.U.
Vitamin C: 3 mg

Soups, Stews, and Salads

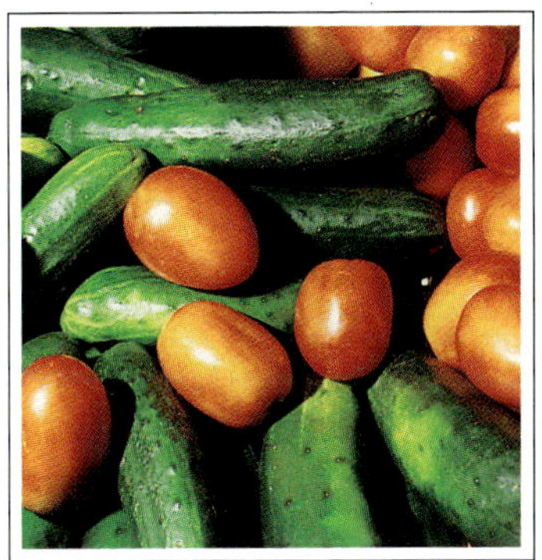
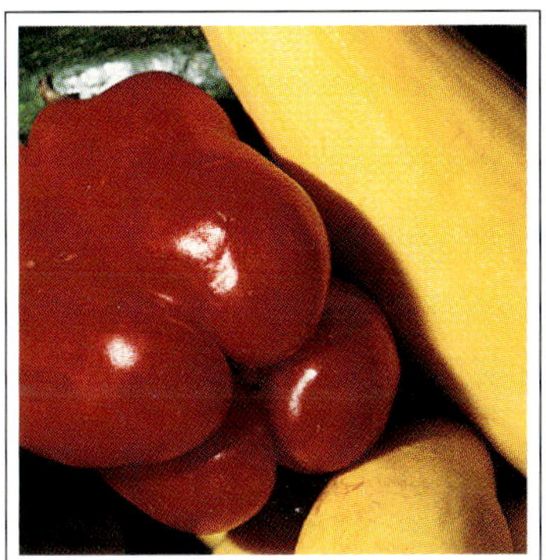
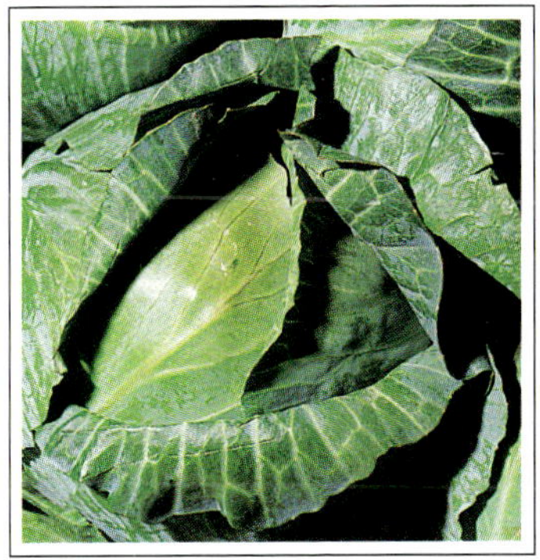
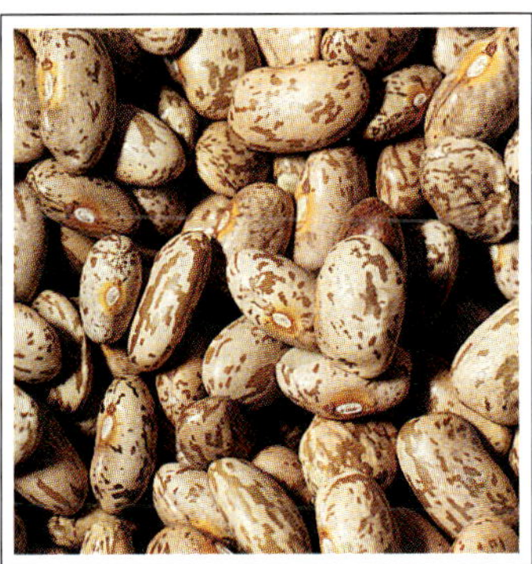

Barley Stew

1 tablespoon Olive Oil

2 pressed cloves of Garlic

1 chopped Onion

1 28 oz. can of Stewed Tomatoes

1 18.5 oz. can of Beef Barley Soup

5 cubes Beef Bouillon

1 cup rinsed Barley

2 shredded Carrots

1/2 cup of cooked Spinach

In a skillet sauté garlic and onion in olive oil. Pour 3 cups of hot water in a soup pot and add bouillon cubes. Add stewed tomatoes, beef barley soup (a brand low in saturated fat), barley, carrots, spinach, garlic and onion to soup pot. Simmer for 45 minutes.

Number of Servings: 6
Nutritional Analysis Per Serving:
Calories: 220
Fat: 5 gm (19%)
Fiber: 3 gm
Cholesterol: 3 mg
Saturated Fat: less than 1 gm
Beta Carotene: 8,800 I.U.
Vitamin C: 30 mg

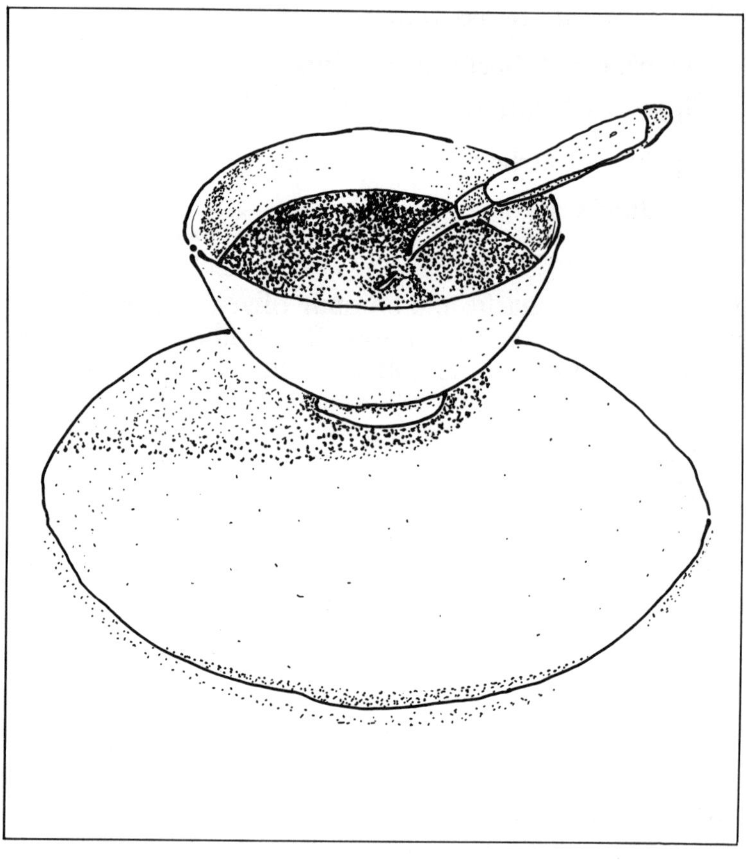

Broccoli Soup

Broccoli Soup

1 bunch of Broccoli

1 cup drained, Non-Fat Yogurt

Dash of Salt and Pepper

Cut broccoli into flowerets and wash in colander. Simmer broccoli for 20 minutes on stove in large soup pot. After broccoli has finished simmering, drain off excess water and allow to cool for 1 hour. After broccoli is cool, place it in a food processor. Using the steel blade attachment, puree the broccoli. When finished, put broccoli in bowl and fold in strained yogurt. Reheat before serving.

Number of Servings: 2
Nutritional Analysis Per Serving:
Calories: 150
Fat: less than 1 gm (5%)
Fiber: 5 gm
Cholesterol: 2 mg
Saturated Fat: less than 1 gm
Beta Carotene: 4,350 I.U.
Vitamin C: 100 mg

Broccoli and Cauliflower Soup

1 bunch of Broccoli

1 bunch of Cauliflower

1 cup drained, Non-Fat Yogurt

Dash of Salt and Pepper

Cut broccoli and cauliflower into flowerets and wash in colander. Simmer both for 20 minutes on stove in large soup pot. After the broccoli and cauliflower have finished simmering, drain off excess water carefully and place in a food processor. Using the steel blade attachment, puree the broccoli and cauliflower. When finished, put in bowl and fold in strained yogurt. Reheat before serving.

Number of Servings: 2
Nutritional Analysis Per Serving:
Calories: 210
Fat: less than 1 gm (3%)
Fiber: 8 gm
Cholesterol: 2 mg
Saturated Fat: less than 1 gm
Beta Carotene: 4,400 I.U.
Vitamin C: 170 mg

Carrot and Rice Soup

2 thinly sliced Leeks

4 peeled and thinly sliced Carrots

1 cup cooked Brown Rice (white rice may also be used)

6 cubes Chicken Bouillon

1 cup drained, Non-Fat Yogurt

In large soup pot combine 7 cups of hot water and chicken bouillon cubes. Bring broth to a rolling boil, then reduce to a simmer. Add leeks and carrots, cook for 15 minutes. Add brown rice and allow to simmer for 15 minutes. Remove from heat, cool for 10 minutes and add yogurt. Stir well.

Number of Servings: 2
Nutritional Analysis Per Serving:
Calories: 300
Fat: 2 gm (6%)
Fiber: 5 gm
Cholesterol: 4 mg
Saturated Fat: less than 1 gm
Beta Carotene: 40,000 I.U.
Vitamin C: 15 mg

Chicken Soup with Pasta and Beans

1 28 oz. can of Stewed Tomatoes

1 15 oz. can of Navy Beans

6 cubes of Chicken Bouillon

1 8 oz. package of short Pasta (or Greek Orzo)

3 shredded Carrots

1 sliced Leek

1 stalk of Celery, chopped

1 pressed clove of Garlic

Dash of Salt and Pepper

In large soup pot, combine 7 cups of hot water and chicken bouillon cubes. Bring broth to a rolling boil, turn down heat and simmer. Add stewed tomatoes and navy beans, allow to simmer for 15 minutes. Add carrots, leek, celery, garlic, salt and pepper. Simmer 15 minutes. Add pasta and cook 8 minutes or until *al dente.*

Number of Servings: 6
Nutritional Analysis Per Serving:
Calories: 220
Fat: less than 1 gm (4%)
Fiber: 3 gm
Cholesterol: less than 1 mg
Saturated Fat: less than 1 gm
Beta Carotene: 11,500 I.U.
Vitamin C: 25 mg

Chicken and Rice Soup

2 skinned, cleaned Chicken Breasts

1 cup cooked Brown Rice (white rice may also be used)

6 cubes Chicken Bouillon

1 chopped, sweet Onion

2 thinly sliced Leeks

1 pressed clove of Garlic

1 tablespoon of Olive Oil

Sauté in skillet olive oil, onion, leeks and garlic. When leeks are clear add chicken breasts. Cook approximately 20 minutes, turning frequently. While chicken is cooking in skillet, prepare broth in large soup pot by combining 7 cups of hot water and chicken bouillon. Bring to rolling boil, then turn down to a simmer. Remove chicken from skillet. Add leeks, onion and garlic to soup pot. Allow chicken to cool for a few minutes, cut into small pieces and add to soup pot. After 10 - 15 minutes, add brown rice and allow to simmer for 15 additional minutes.

Number of Servings: 2
Nutritional Analysis Per Serving:
Calories: 460
Fat: 13 gm (25%)
Fiber: 4 gm
Cholesterol: 100 mg
Saturated Fat: 2 gm
Beta Carotene: 25 I.U.
Vitamin C: 8 mg

Chicken and Garbanzo Bean Stew

1 skinned, cleaned Chicken Breast

1 15 oz. can of Garbanzo Beans

5 cubes Chicken Bouillon

3 shredded Carrots

2 sliced Leeks

1 pressed clove of Garlic

1 tablespoon Olive Oil

Dash of Salt and Pepper

Sauté in skillet olive oil, leeks and garlic. When leeks are clear add chicken breast. Cook approximately 20 minutes, turning frequently. While chicken is cooking in skillet, prepare broth in large soup pot by combining 7 cups of hot water and chicken bouillon. Bring to rolling boil, then turn down to a simmer, add garbanzo beans. Remove chicken from skillet. Add carrots, leeks and garlic to soup pot. Allow chicken to cool for a few minutes, cut into small pieces and add to soup pot. Salt and pepper to taste. Simmer for 1 hour.

Number of Servings: 4
Nutritional Analysis Per Serving:
Calories: 270
Fat: 7 gm (20%)
Fiber: 7 gm
Cholesterol: 25 mg
Saturated Fat: 1 gm
Beta Carotene: 15,000 I.U.
Vitamin C: 5 mg

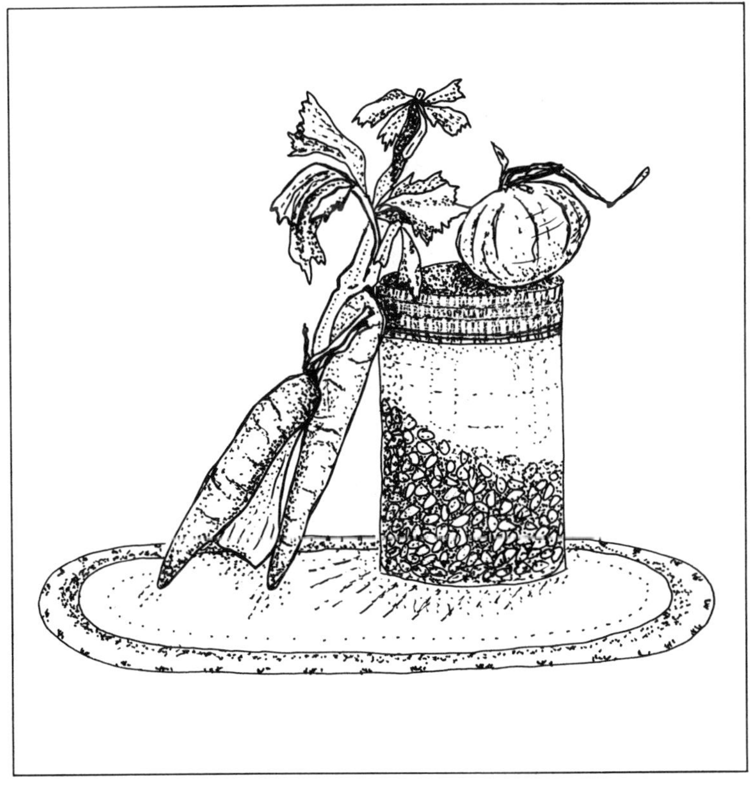

Chili

Chili

1 chopped Onion

1 chopped Green Pepper

3 shredded Carrots

2 pressed cloves of Garlic

1 15 oz. can of Kidney Beans

1 15 oz. can of Pinto Beans

3 15 oz. cans of Tomato Sauce

1 6 oz. can of Tomato Paste

1 tablespoon Chili Pepper

In large soup pot combine all ingredients. Be sure to wash beans in a colander first. Allow to simmer 2 to 3 hours.

Number of Servings: 6
Nutritional Analysis Per Serving:
Calories: 300
Fat: 1 gm (3%)
Fiber: 14 gm
Cholesterol: -0-
Saturated Fat: less than 1 gm
Beta Carotene: 13,500 I.U.
Vitamin C: 65 mg

Cod and Rice Stew

4 cooked Cod Fish Fillets

4 shredded Carrots

2 cubed Potatoes

2 chopped Onions

1 15 oz. can of Tomato Sauce

1 6 oz. can of Tomato Paste

1 tablespoon Olive Oil

2 pressed cloves of Garlic

2 sprigs of Parsley

In soup pot, combine tomato sauce, tomato paste, olive oil, garlic and onions; bring to a simmer. Add 4 cups of warm water, potatoes and carrots. Allow to simmer for 45 minutes. Add parsley and cod. Simmer an additional 15 minutes.

Number of Servings: 6
Nutritional Analysis Per Serving:
Calories: 300
Fat: 6 gm (18%)
Fiber: 1 gm
Cholesterol: 27 mg
Saturated Fat: 1 gm
Beta Carotene: 15,000 I.U.
Vitamin C: 60 mg

Corn Chowder, Southern Style

10 ears Corn on the Cob

2 cups of Skim Milk

1 tablespoon Sugar

Butter Buds

Serve with: Scallions, Radishes and Green Pepper

Over a large bowl, with a very sharp knife, cut just the top off of each kernel of corn. Then taking a spoon, scrape downward on the cob to remove the corn germ. Spray a skillet with non-stick spray and pour in the prepared corn. Add skim milk. Be sure to keep the heat low and stir very frequently. The starch from the corn will have a tendency to stick very easily. When corn is almost finished (after about 10 minutes) add sugar and stir well. Remove from heat. Sprinkle with Butter Buds. Serve with garnishes suggested above.

Number of Servings: 4
Nutritional Analysis Per Serving:
Calories: 266
Fat: 2 gm (7%)
Fiber: 1 gm
Cholesterol: 2 mg
Saturated Fat: less than 1 gm
Beta Carotene: 675 I.U.
Vitamin C: 15 mg

Corn Chowder, Quick and Easy

1 large bag of frozen Corn

1 cup of Skim Milk

3 shredded Carrots

1 diced Green Pepper

1 diced Red Pepper

Butter Buds

In sauce pan combine corn and milk. Heat for 5 minutes over low heat, stirring often. Add carrots, green pepper and red pepper. Cook an additional 5 minutes. Sprinkle with Butter Buds and serve.

Number of Servings: 4
Nutritional Analysis Per Serving:
Calories: 188
Fat: trace
Fiber: 8 gm
Cholesterol: 1 mg
Saturated Fat: trace
Beta Carotene: 16,500 I.U.
Vitamin C: 70 mg

Gazpacho

1 28 oz. can of Pear Tomatoes

2 peeled Cucumber

2 diced Red Peppers

1 diced Green Pepper

2 chopped Onions (1 red, 1 yellow)

3 pressed cloves of Garlic

1 tablespoon Olive Oil

1/2 cup Red Vinegar

Dash of Cumin (to taste)

Dash of Salt

Put aside a small portion of the prepared cucumbers, red peppers, green pepper and onions. In a food processor combine the remaining ingredients, mix extremely well. Allow to cool in refrigerator for 2 hours before serving. If this is not possible, add 4 cubes of ice and stir until cubes have melted. Place in serving bowls, sprinkle with vegetables set aside earlier. A piece of cut parsley may be added to each bowl as garnishment.

Number of Servings: 4
Nutritional Analysis Per Serving:
Calories: 100
Fat: 3 gm (27%)
Fiber: 4 gm
Cholesterol: -0-
Saturated Fat: less than 1 gm
Beta Carotene: 5,000 I.U.
Vitamin C: 110 mg

Hearty Lentil Soup

2 cups dried Lentils

3 15 oz. cans of Tomato Sauce

3 shredded Carrots

1 chopped Onion

Allow lentils to simmer in three cups of water for approximately 1 hour. Carefully drain lentils through colander. In soup pot, combine tomato sauce, carrots, onion and lentils. Cook on low heat for 1 hour.

Number of Servings: 6
Nutritional Analysis Per Serving:
Calories: 242
Fat: less than 1 gm (2.4%)
Fiber: 3 gm
Cholesterol: -0-
Saturated Fat: less than 1 gm
Beta Carotene: 11,000 I.U.
Vitamin C: 35 mg

Navy Bean Soup

2 cups dried Navy Beans

3 15 oz. cans of Tomato Sauce

3 shredded Carrots

1 chopped Onion

Allow beans to simmer in 4 cups of water for approximately 1 and 1/2 hours. Carefully drain beans through colander. In soup pot, combine tomato sauce, carrots, onion and beans. Cook on low heat for 1 hour.

Number of Servings: 6
Nutritional Analysis Per Serving:
Calories: 250
Fat: less than 1 gm (1.2%)
Fiber: 5 gm
Cholesterol: -0-
Saturated Fat: -0-
Beta Carotene: 11,000 I.U.
Vitamin C: 35 mg

Pasta and Garbanzo Bean Soup

1 8 oz. package of short Macaroni

1 15 oz. can of Garbanzo Beans

1 tablespoon Olive Oil

3 pressed cloves of Garlic

2 cubes of Chicken Bouillon

Salt and Pepper to taste

In large soup pot bring 7 cups of water to a boil then turn down. Add chicken bouillon cubes. Add prepared garbanzo beans. Add olive oil and garlic. Simmer for 3 to 4 hours. Be sure not to cover the soup pot while cooking or the beans will not cook properly. Ten minutes before serving soup add macaroni.

Number of Servings: 6
Nutritional Analysis Per Serving:
Calories: 150
Fat: 3 gm (18%)
Fiber: 6 gm
Cholesterol: trace
Saturated Fat: less than 1 gm
Beta Carotene: trace
Vitamin C: -0-

Potato and Shallot Soup

5 Potatoes

3 chopped Shallots

1 pressed clove of Garlic

4 cups of Skim Milk

Salt and Pepper to taste

Butter Buds to taste

In skillet sauté shallots and garlic until clear. While waiting, peel and cut potatoes into cubes. Place in large pot of boiling water. Boil for 20 minutes. Drain and allow to cool. Put in food processor and cut with steel blade, slowly adding skim milk until smooth and creamy. Blend in garlic and shallots slowly. Add butter buds, salt and pepper to taste.

Number of Servings: 6
Nutritional Analysis Per Serving:
Calories: 150
Fat: trace
Fiber: 5 gm
Cholesterol: 3 mg
Saturated Fat: less than 1 gm
Beta Carotene: 333 I.U.
Vitamin C: 53 mg

Summer Vegetable Medley

1 Onion

1 Eggplant

1 Green Pepper

1 Zucchini

1 28 oz. can of Stewed Tomatoes

3 pressed cloves of Garlic

1 tablespoon Olive Oil

Dash of Salt and Pepper

Cut onion into quarters. To prepare eggplant, cut in half lengthwise then slice each half into thin slices. Cut green pepper into small cubes. Slice zucchini into thin slices. In large soup pot, slowly heat olive oil and sauté garlic. Add tomatoes and remaining ingredients already prepared as noted above. Cook over low heat for 45 minutes to 1 hour. This is a dish that tastes even better if served the following day.

Number of Servings: 6
Nutritional Analysis Per Serving:
Calories: 75
Fat: 2.5 gm (30%)
Fiber: 6 gm
Cholesterol: -0-
Saturated Fat: less than 1 gm
Beta Carotene: 1,600 I.U.
Vitamin C: 37 mg

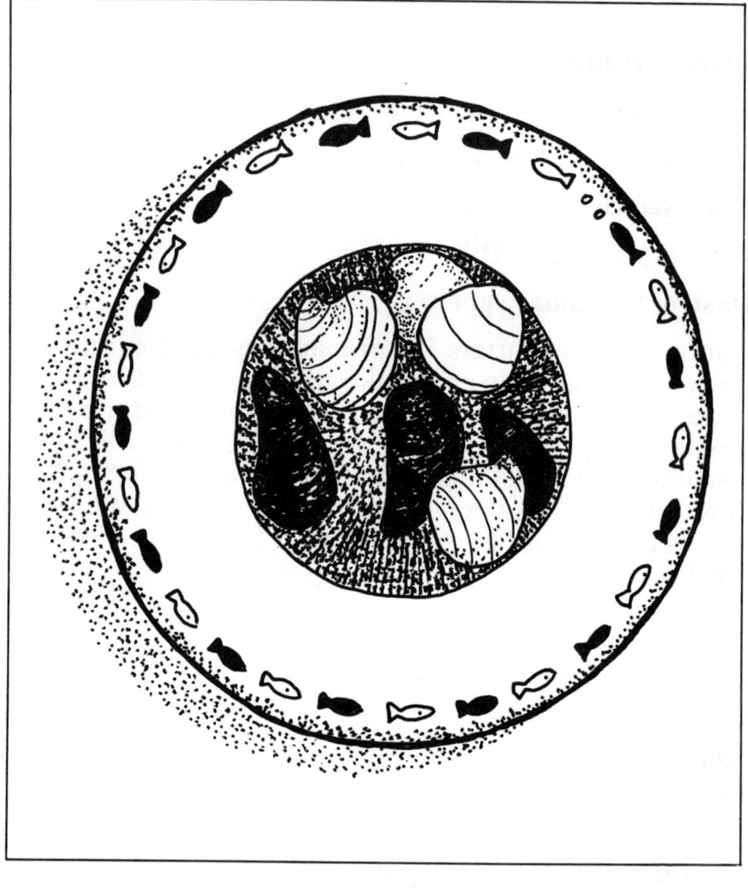

Seafood Soup with Pasta

Seafood Soup with Pasta

1 pound Shellfish (clams, mussels, etc.)

1 pound Fish (bass, halibut, etc.)

3 shredded Carrots

1 chopped Onion

1 diced stalk of Celery

1 15 oz. can of Tomato Sauce

2 teaspoons Olive Oil

1 8 oz. package of short Pasta

Dash of Salt and Pepper

In large pot simmer fish, carrots, onion and celery with a dash of salt and pepper for 2 hours, be sure there is at least 4 cups of water. Allow to simmer until liquid becomes a broth, taking on the fish flavors. While the large pot simmers, begin to cook the shellfish by placing them in a pot of gently boiling water. When the shells have opened they are done. Remove the shells, set meat aside. When fish is finished cooking, make sure there are at least 4 cups of water in the large pot, add tomato sauce, olive oil and pasta, cook for 5 minutes. Add shellfish and pasta, cook another 5 minutes.

Number of Servings: 8
Nutritional Analysis Per Serving:
Calories: 156
Fat: 4 gm (20%)
Fiber: 1 gm
Cholesterol: 57 mg
Saturated Fat: less than 1 gm
Beta Carotene: 812 I.U.
Vitamin C: 5 mg

Split Pea Soup

4 diced Potatoes

1/2 pound Split Peas

4 shredded Carrots

1 chopped sweet Onion

2 pressed cloves of Garlic

In a large pot cook peas in approximately 6 cups of water for 20 - 30 minutes or until they become very soft. Add potatoes, carrots, onion and garlic. Cook for 1 and a half hours. Make sure water level remains constant. If you would like to try a variation, add 3-4 tablespoons of curry powder when beginning to cook split peas.

Number of Servings: 6
Nutritional Analysis Per Serving:
Calories: 200
Fat: trace
Fiber: 8 gm
Cholesterol: -0-
Saturated Fat: -0-
Beta Carotene: 13,000 I.U.
Vitamin C: 24 mg

Vegetable Stew

5 peeled, sliced Potatoes

5 shredded Carrots

1 bunch of Spinach, chopped

2 cups cut Green Beans

2 15 oz. cans of Tomato Sauce

Oregano, Salt and Pepper to taste

Prepare vegetables, mix well, place in soup pot. Add tomato sauce, 2 cups of water and spices. Simmer for 3 hours.

Number of Servings: 4
Nutritional Analysis Per Serving:
Calories: 320
Fat: trace
Fiber: 6 gm
Cholesterol: -0-
Saturated Fat: -0-
Beta Carotene: 30,000 I.U.
Vitamin C: 100 mg

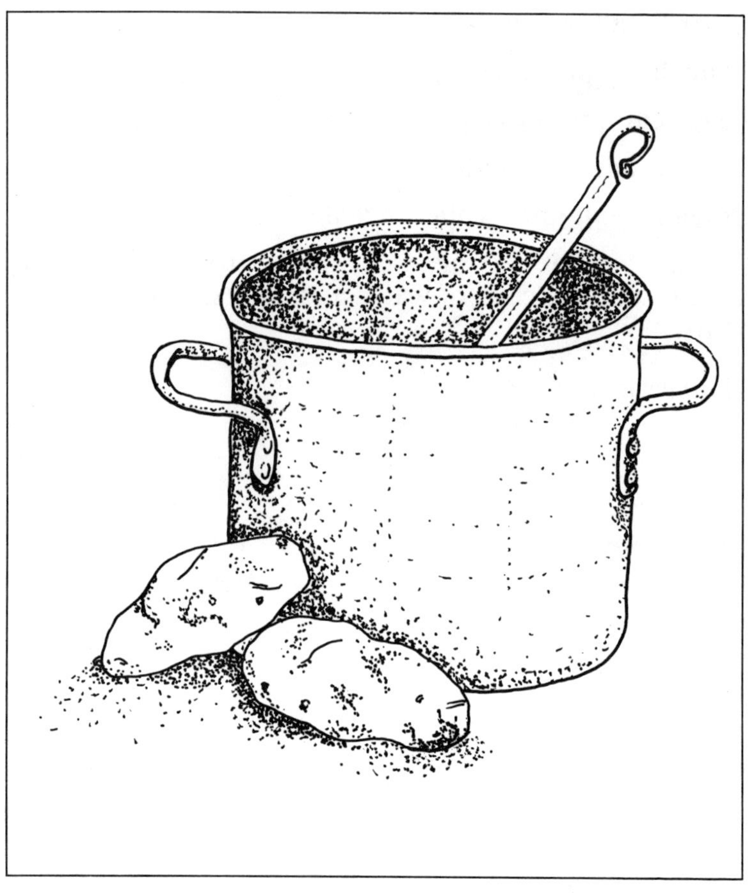

Vichyssoise

Vichyssoise

4 cups peeled, cubed Potatoes

2 cups chopped Onions

1 sliced Leek

1 cup drained Non-Fat Yogurt

Skim Milk (as needed)

Salt and Pepper to taste

Bring 4 cups of water to rolling boil. Add potatoes, cook for 20 minutes. While potatoes are boiling, sauté onions and leek in skillet. When potatoes have finished, drain and allow to cool. In food processor, combine potatoes, onions and leek along with yogurt. Add skim milk as needed, very carefully, to achieve a rich, creamy consistency. Salt and pepper to taste.

Number of Servings: 4
Nutritional Analysis Per Serving:
Calories: 170
Fat: trace
Fiber: 2 gm
Cholesterol: 1 mg
Saturated Fat: less than 1 gm
Beta Carotene: 65 I.U.
Vitamin C: 32 mg

Broccoli Salad

1 head Broccoli

2 tablespoons Olive Oil

1 cup Red Wine Vinegar

2 tablespoons Italian Seasonings

Steam broccoli flowerets for 10 minutes. Combine olive oil, vinegar and seasonings. When broccoli is finished steaming, place in bowl and cover completely with seasonings, allow to marinate for at least 20 minutes at room temperature. Serve or chill for later use. Suggested vegetable garnishes include: tomato, cauliflower, red onion, black olives, green and red peppers.

Number of Servings: 4
Nutritional Analysis Per Serving:
Calories: 35
Fat: 2 gm (51%)
Fiber: 3 gm
Cholesterol: -0-
Saturated Fat: less than 1 gm
Beta Carotene: 1,100 I.U.
Vitamin C: 50 mg

Bulgur Wheat Salad

2 cups Bulgur Wheat

1 grated Carrot

4 tablespoons Lemon Juice

1/2 bunch of Ground Parsley

1 tablespoon Ground Mint

1 tablespoon Olive Oil

Bring 2 cups of water to a rolling boil. Pour over bulgur wheat (in heat resistant bowl) and allow to sit for 10 minutes. The easiest, and perhaps best way to prepare the parsley and mint is to grind them in a food processor. Drain any excess water from the bowl of wheat after 10 minutes. Add ground seasonings, olive oil, lemon juice and carrot. Chill and serve.

Number of Servings: 8
Nutritional Analysis Per Serving:
Calories: 170
Fat: 2.5 gm (13%)
Fiber: 3 gm
Cholesterol: -0-
Saturated Fat: less than 1 gm
Beta Carotene: 3,000 I.U.
Vitamin C: 1 mg

Chinese Cabbage

1 chopped head of Cabbage

10 tablespoons Salt

3 cups White Vinegar

1 cup Sugar

1 teaspoon Cayenne Pepper

Liberally salt cabbage in a colander and set aside for a half hour. Rinse salt out completely (for a minimum of 10 minutes) then set aside. Dissolve sugar in simmering vinegar. Place cabbage in air tight container. Allow vinegar/sugar mixture to cool. Poor over cabbage, covering completely. Carefully add cayenne pepper and mix thoroughly. Seal container and allow to marinate in refrigerator for three days.

Number of Servings: 12
Nutritional Analysis Per Serving:
Calories: 12
Fat: -0-
Fiber: trace
Cholesterol: -0-
Saturated Fat: -0-
Beta Carotene: -0-
Vitamin C: 10 mg

Old Fashion Coleslaw

1 head shredded Cabbage

1 cup Skim Milk

3 shredded Carrots

1/2 cup Reduced-Fat Mayonnaise

3 tablespoons Sugar

1/2 cup Vinegar

Salt and Pepper to taste

In large bowl combine all ingredients. Place in air tight container and cool in refrigerator.

Number of Servings: 12
Nutritional Analysis Per Serving:
Calories: 50
Fat: 1 gm (18%)
Fiber: 2 gm
Cholesterol: 2 mg
Saturated Fat: less than 1 gm
Beta Carotene: 5,000 I.U.
Vitamin C: 10 mg

Curried Garbanzo Beans

1 15 oz. can of Garbanzo Beans

1 tablespoon Curry

1 chopped Onion

2 pressed cloves of Garlic

1 chopped Tomato

2 teaspoons Olive Oil

1 chopped Scallion

In a skillet sauté onion, garlic and olive oil on low heat. In a medium bowl combine washed and drained garbanzo beans, curry and tomato. Add onion mixture. Allow to marinate overnight in air tight container. Top with scallions before serving.

Number of Servings: 4
Nutritional Analysis Per Serving:
Calories: 175
Fat: 4 gm (21%)
Fiber: 7 gm
Cholesterol: -0-
Saturated Fat: less than 1 gm
Beta Carotene: 2,000 I.U.
Vitamin C: 12 mg

Hearty Salad

3 cups Green Beans

1 cup shredded Carrots

2 cups Broccoli flowerets

2 cups Cauliflower flowerets

2 chopped Scallions

2 teaspoons Italian Seasonings

1 tablespoon Olive Oil

Cut ends from green beans and steam for 2 minutes. Add broccoli and cauliflower, cut into flowerets, and cook for an additional 3 - 5 minutes. Vegetables should be tender yet crunchy. Remove from heat and rinse with cool water. Drain well. Place in large bowl and stir in remaining ingredients. For additional taste and crunch, add 1 tablespoon toasted sesame seeds and mix well.

Number of Servings: 12
Nutritional Analysis Per Serving:
Calories: 40
Fat: 1 gm (27%)
Fiber: 4 gm
Cholesterol: -0-
Saturated Fat: less than 1 gm
Beta Carotene: 2,250 I.U.
Vitamin C: 35 mg

Lima Bean Salad

1 15 oz. can of Lima Beans

1 chopped sweet Onion

1 stalk of Celery, chopped

1 tablespoon Olive Oil

1 teaspoon Italian Seasonings

Rinse and drain lima beans. Combine all ingredients above in a bowl. Place in air tight container and cool.

Number of Servings: 4
Nutritional Analysis Per Serving:
Calories: 140
Fat: 4 gm (25%)
Fiber: 4 gm
Cholesterol: -0-
Saturated Fat: less than 1 gm
Beta Carotene: 162 I.U.
Vitamin C: 15 mg

Macaroni Salad

1 12 oz. package of mixed Macaroni (green, orange and yellow)

1 tablespoon finely chopped sweet Onion

1/2 cup Reduced-Fat Mayonnaise

1 tablespoon of Feta Cheese, crumbled

2 sliced Black Olives

Prepare macaroni as indicated on package. Drain and cool. Mix all ingredients in large bowl. Before serving, garnish top with black olives.

Number of Servings: 6
Nutritional Analysis Per Serving:
Calories: 216
Fat: 5 gm (19%)
Fiber: 2 gm
Cholesterol: 8 mg
Saturated Fat: 1 gm
Beta Carotene: 12 I.U.
Vitamin C: trace

New Potato Salad

15 New Potatoes

1 bunch finely chopped Scallions

1/4 cup Reduced-Fat Mayonnaise

1/2 cup chopped Celery

1 tablespoon Low-Cal Italian Salad Dressing

Salt and Pepper to taste

Wash and cube potatoes; it is not necessary to peel. Bring water to a rolling boil, place potatoes in water and cook for 15 minutes. Drain potatoes in colander and allow to cool. Combine all ingredients in large bowl and mix well. Serve warm or store in air tight container and place in refrigerator.

Number of Servings: 8
Nutritional Analysis Per Serving:
Calories: 135
Fat: 2 gm (10%)
Fiber: 3 gm
Cholesterol: 2 mg
Saturated Fat: less than 1 gm
Beta Carotene: 6 I.U.
Vitamin C: 33 mg

Rice Salad

3 cups cooked long grain Rice, cooled

1 1/2 cups cubed, cooked Beets

2 finely chopped Scallion tips (white portion)

2 black or green pitted, chopped Greek Olives

1 tablespoon Olive Oil

1 tablespoon Red Wine Vinegar

1 tablespoon Reduced-Fat Mayonnaise

Place the rice, beets, scallion and olives in a large bowl and stir together. Add olive oil, vinegar and mayonnaise. Mix very well until completely combined. Add salt and pepper, if needed.

Number of Servings: 6
Nutritional Analysis Per Serving:
Calories: 131
Fat: 3 gm (20%)
Fiber: 1 gm
Cholesterol: 1 mg
Saturated Fat: less than 1 gm
Beta Carotene: 2,100 I.U.
Vitamin C: 4 mg

Summer Rice Salad

3 cups long grain Rice, cooled

1 cup chopped Scallions

1 cup chopped Celery

1 thinly sliced Cucumber

1 cup thinly sliced Radish

1 cup shredded Carrots

2 tablespoons Olive Oil

1 tablespoon Red Wine Vinegar

Dash of Salt and Pepper

Put rice in a large bowl. In a small container, mix together olive oil and vinegar. Pour on rice a little at a time, tossing with a metal fork. Toss in ingredients one at a time - tossing between each addition. When mixture is completely tossed together, salt and pepper to taste.

Number of Servings: 6
Nutritional Analysis Per Serving:
Calories: 130
Fat: 2 gm (16%)
Fiber: 2 gm
Cholesterol: -0-
Saturated Fat: less than 1 gm
Beta Carotene: 5,600 I.U.
Vitamin C: 8 mg

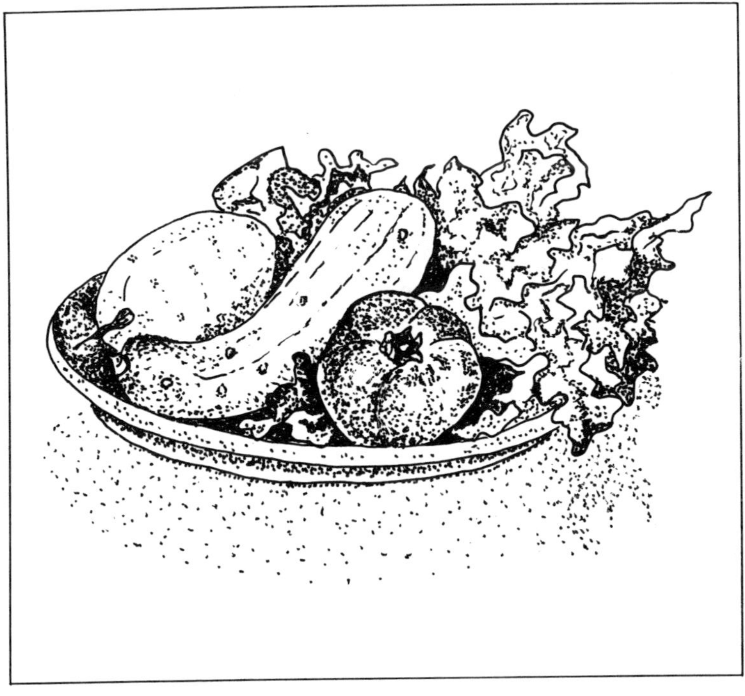

Simply Salad

Simply Salad

1 head torn Lettuce leaves, any type

2 Tomatoes, cut into wedges

1/4 cup sliced Purple Onion

1/4 cup sliced sweet Onion

1/2 cup Bean Sprouts

1/4 cup chopped Green Peppers

1 cup shredded Carrot

1 thinly sliced Cucumber

Toss all ingredients lightly in large bowl. Be sure to wash all ingredients well before beginning.

Number of Servings: 6
Nutritional Analysis Per Serving:
Calories: 27
Fat: -0-
Fiber: 1 gm
Cholesterol: -0-
Saturated Fat: -0-
Beta Carotene: 6,000 I.U.
Vitamin C: 31 mg

Shallot and Garbanzo Bean Salad

1 head of torn Spinach

2 Tomatoes, cut into wedges

1 15 oz. can of Garbanzo Beans

3 thinly sliced Shallots

1 cup shredded Carrot

1 thinly sliced Cucumber

Toss all ingredients lightly in a large bowl. Be sure to wash all ingredients well before beginning.

Number of Servings: 8
Nutritional Analysis Per Serving:
Calories: 85
Fat: 1 gm (10%)
Fiber: 2 gm
Cholesterol: -0-
Saturated Fat: less than 1 gm
Beta Carotene: 5,000 I.U.
Vitamin C: 12 mg

Tabouli

1 cup dry, cracked Wheat

1/2 cup chopped Parsley

1 teaspoon chopped Fresh Mint

2 diced Tomatoes

2 thinly sliced Scallions

1 teaspoon Olive Oil

4 tablespoons Lemon Juice

Soak wheat in 2 cups warm water for 20 minutes, drain well. Toss moist wheat with parsley, mint, tomato and scallion. Add olive oil and lemon juice, mix well. May be garnished with a sprig of parsley and a few olives if desired.

Number of Servings: 6
Nutritional Analysis Per Serving:
Calories: 132
Fat: 1 gm (7%)
Fiber: 2 gm
Cholesterol: -0-
Saturated Fat: less than 1 gm
Beta Carotene: 633 I.U.
Vitamin C: 7 mg

Bean Salad

1 15 oz. can of each: Lima, Red Kidney, Yellow Wax and/or Green Beans
1 chopped Green Pepper
1 shredded Carrot
1/3 thinly chopped Purple Onion
1 package of Italian Seasonings
2 tablespoons Sugar
1/2 cup Red Wine Vinegar

Wash and drain beans well. In large bowl combine all ingredients and toss gently. Allow to marinate overnight.

Number of Servings: 12
Nutritional Analysis Per Serving:
Calories: 100
Fat: less than 1 gm (3%)
Fiber: 8 gm
Cholesterol: -0-
Saturated Fat: less than 1 gm
Beta Carotene: 2,000 I.U.
Vitamin C: 15 mg

Tropical Salad

2 peeled and cut Oranges

2 cups crushed Pineapple

3 grated Carrots

4 tablespoons Raisins

1/2 cup Non-Fat Yogurt

2 tablespoons Orange Preserves

3 tablespoons Lemon Juice

In large bowl combine oranges, pineapple, carrots and raisins, mix well. In separate bowl combine yogurt, orange preserves and lemon juice, stir until well mixed. Place fruit in air-tight container, pour topping over fruit and seal.

Number of Servings: 6
Nutritional Analysis Per Serving:
Calories: 105
Fat: less than 1 gm (3%)
Fiber: 2 gm
Cholesterol: -0-
Saturated Fat: less than 1 gm
Beta Carotene: 10,000 I.U.
Vitamin C: 40 mg

White Bean Salad

1/2 cup Bulgur Wheat

1 1/2 cups cooked White Beans

1 cup diced Tomatoes

2 thinly chopped Scallions

1 cup chopped Parsley

2 tablespoons Lemon Juice

1 tablespoon Olive Oil

Soak bulgur wheat in 1/2 cup of hot water for 20 minutes, drain well and place in mixing bowl. Add beans, tomato, scallions and parsley, mix well. Add lemon juice and olive oil and mix thoroughly. Allow to marinate overnight.

Number of Servings: 6
Nutritional Analysis Per Serving:
Calories: 130
Fat: 3 gm (20%)
Fiber: 3 gm
Cholesterol: -0-
Saturated Fat: less than 1 gm
Beta Carotene: 500 I.U.
Vitamin C: 10 mg

Winter Fresh Fruit Salad

2 sliced tart Red Apples

1 sliced Green Apple

2 peeled, sectioned Oranges

1/2 sectioned Grapefruit

1 peeled, sliced Pear

1/2 cup Raisins

1 cup Orange Juice

1 tablespoon Lemon Juice

1 8 oz. container of Fruit Yogurt

In large bowl combine all of the above ingredients except fruit yogurt. Mix well. Store in air-tight container. Serve with fruit yogurt as topping.

Number of Servings: 6
Nutritional Analysis Per Serving:
Calories: 188
Fat: trace
Fiber: 28 gm
Cholesterol: -0-
Saturated Fat: less than 1 gm
Beta Carotene: 350 I.U.
Vitamin C: 58 mg

The Main Course

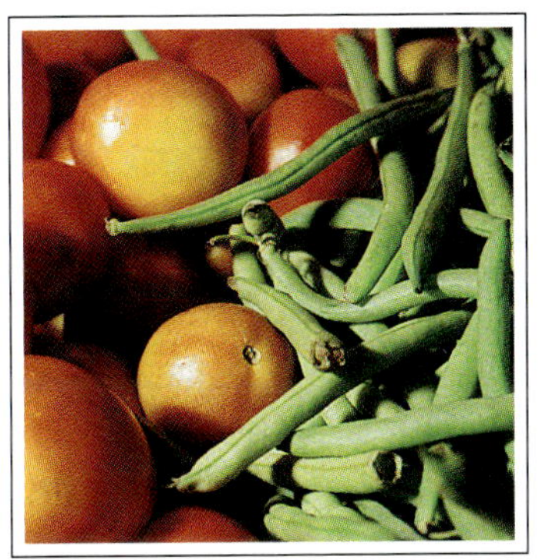

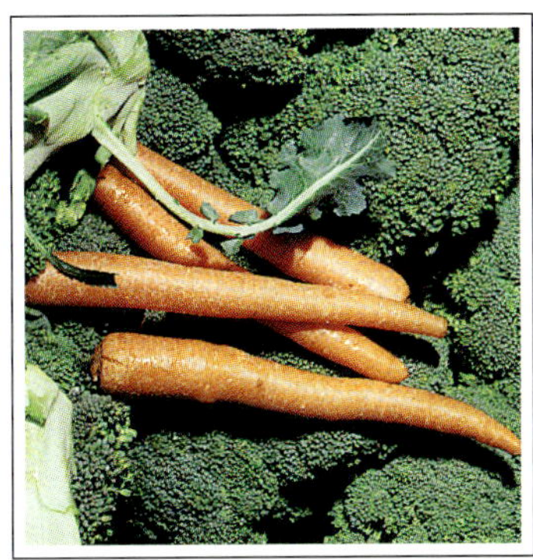

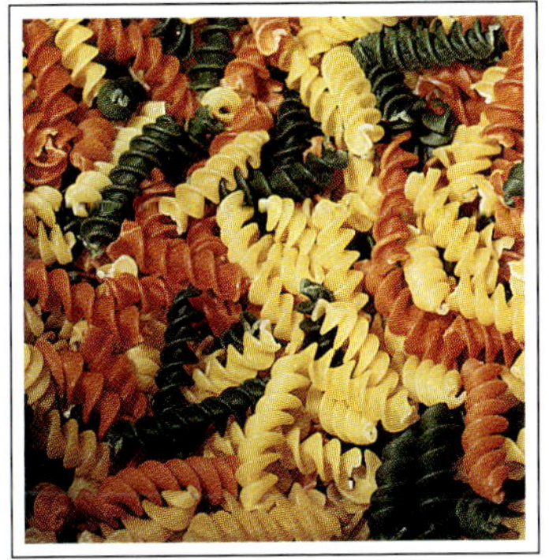

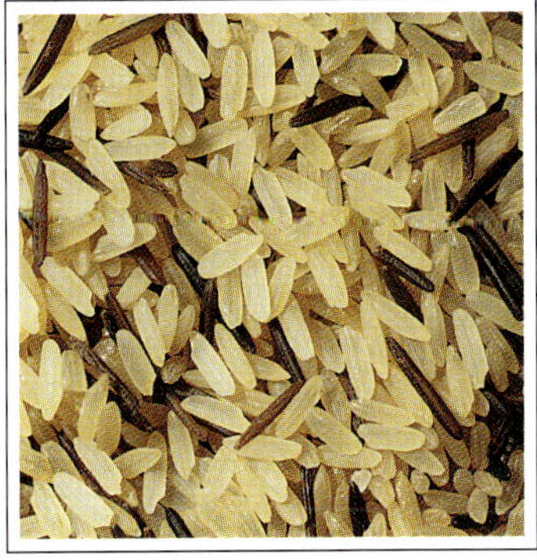

Broiled Shrimp

1 pound Jumbo Shrimp

1/2 cup White Wine

1 tablespoon Olive Oil

1 tablespoon Oregano

3 pressed cloves of Garlic

Wash and drain shrimp in colander. In a large shallow dish mix together white wine, olive oil, oregano and garlic. Allow shrimp to marinate for 30 minutes in refrigerator. Drain shrimp in colander. Spread shrimp on baking sheet in single layer. Broil for 5 to 10 minutes or until shrimp turns bright pink.

Number of Servings: 4
Nutritional Analysis Per Serving:
Calories: 183
Fat: 5 gm (23%)
Fiber: -0-
Cholesterol: 170 mg
Saturated Fat: less than 1 gm
Beta Carotene: 66 I.U.
Vitamin C: -0-

Baked Fish

6 Cod Fish Fillets

1 tablespoon Olive Oil

1 tablespoon Thyme

Dash of Paprika

Dash of Salt and Pepper

Wash fish and pat dry with paper towels. Place fish in bottom of shallow baking dish sprayed with non-stick spray. Brush each fillet with olive oil, then sprinkle with thyme, paprika, salt and pepper. Bake uncovered in 450 degree oven for 20 - 30 minutes. Fish is finished cooking when it flakes easily when pricked with fork.

Number of Servings: 6
Nutritional Analysis Per Serving:
Calories: 106
Fat: 1 gm (12%)
Fiber: -0-
Cholesterol: 57 mg
Saturated Fat: less than 1 gm
Beta Carotene: 125 I.U.
Vitamin C: -0-

Fish Oriental

6 Cod Fish Fillets

1 chopped Green Pepper

1 chopped Red Pepper

1 8 oz. can of crushed Pineapple

2 tablespoons Soy Sauce

2 tablespoons Corn Starch

Wash and drain fish in colander. Cut fish into strips. Sprinkle fish with cornstarch and set aside. Spray skillet with non-stick spray. Sauté peppers, pineapple and soy sauce over low heat. When mixture begins to thicken, add fish and cook for 5 minutes.

Number of Servings: 6
Nutritional Analysis Per Serving:
Calories: 125
Fat: 1 gm (10%)
Fiber: less than 1 gm
Cholesterol: 78 mg
Saturated Fat: less than 1 gm
Beta Carotene: 124 I.U.
Vitamin C: 43 mg

Corn Meal "Fried" Fish

6 Cod Fish Fillets

2 cups Corn Meal

3 tablespoons Skim Milk

2 Egg Whites

Dash of Salt and Pepper

Wash and drain fish well. Put milk and egg whites in shallow bowl and whisk. Place fish in bowl for a couple of minutes. Put corn meal, salt and pepper in brown paper bag. Place one piece of fish in bag at a time and shake. Pan fry fish in skillet (preferably cast iron) with non-stick spray. Allow fish to cook for at least 10 minutes on each side over medium heat.

Number of Servings: 6
Nutritional Analysis Per Serving:
Calories: 166
Fat: 2 gm (10%)
Fiber: less than 1 gm
Cholesterol: 78 mg
Saturated Fat: less than 1 gm
Beta Carotene: 117 I.U.
Vitamin C: -0-

Pan "Fried" Fish

6 Cod Fish Fillets

1 package of Butter Buds

(prepared according to package directions)

Dash of Salt and Pepper

Wash and drain fish well. Prepare Butter Buds in shallow bowl according to directions then add salt and pepper. Place fish in bowl for a couple of minutes. Pan fry fish in skillet (preferably cast iron) with non-stick spray Allow fish to cook for at least 10 minutes on each side over medium heat.

Number of Servings: 6
Nutritional Analysis Per Serving:
Calories: 135
Fat: 1 gm (8%)
Fiber: -0-
Cholesterol: 80 mg
Saturated Fat: less than 1 gm
Beta Carotene: 40 I.U.
Vitamin C: -0-

Pan Smoked Salmon

6 Salmon Steaks

1/4 cup all purpose Flour

3 tablespoons of Olive Oil, to be used as needed

3/4 teaspoon Thyme

1 bunch Thyme

1 bunch Rosemary

2 tablespoons Whole Black Peppercorns

1 teaspoon grated Lemon Rind

Salt and Pepper to taste

In mixing bowl stir together flour, thyme, salt and pepper. Pour mixture into small brown paper bag. Gently shake salmon steaks in bag of flour mixture one at a time. Sauté salmon in olive oil coated pan until at least half done. While salmon is cooking, soak thyme, rosemary and peppercorns in water for 15 minutes and then set aside. Remove salmon, wipe skillet, but do not thoroughly clean it. Pour more olive oil in skillet until standing 1/4 inch in bottom. Turn heat up and allow skillet to heat until slightly smoking. Place peppercorns, thyme, rosemary in bottom of skillet. Place rack over herbs and arrange salmon steaks on rack. Cover skillet and allow to smoke for about 15 minutes or until fish is done. When finished remove from skillet and garnish with lemon rind. Please be very careful in preparing this dish.

If you wish to prepare a creamy topping one can be made using reduced-fat mayonnaise and finely chopped relish.

Number of Servings: 6
Nutritional Analysis Per Serving:
Calories: 265
Fat: 13 gm (45%)
Fiber: -0-
Cholesterol: 80 mg
Saturated Fat: 2.5 gm
Beta Carotene: 416 I.U.
Vitamin C: -0-

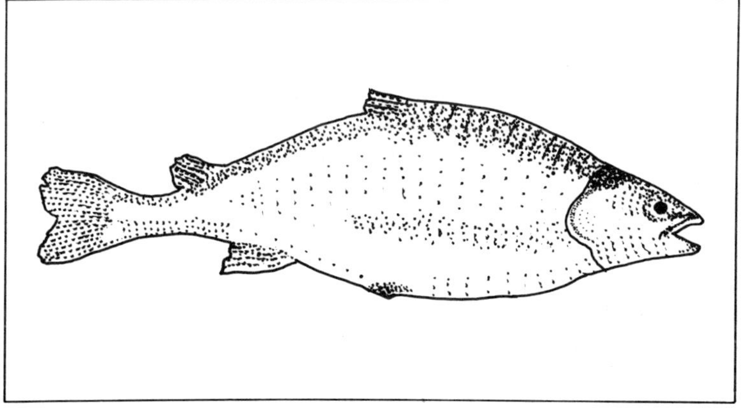

Spinach and Brown Rice Casserole

2 cups cooked long grain Brown Rice

2 10 oz. packages of Spinach

2 chopped Shallots

1 pressed clove of Garlic

1 teaspoon Olive Oil

In a large saucepan sauté olive oil, garlic and shallots over medium heat until clear. Stir in rice, salt and pepper. Slowly add 2 1/2 cups of water. Bring to a boil, cover and allow to simmer on low heat for 30 minutes. Stir in spinach which has been trimmed, washed, drained, chopped and cooked. Cover pan and allow to cook for 10 more minutes or until liquid has been completely absorbed. If rice is not yet tender add a little more hot water and continue to cook. Put into bowl and fluff with fork.

Number of Servings: 4
Nutritional Analysis Per Serving:
Calories: 165
Fat: 1.5 gm (8%)
Fiber: 5 gm
Cholesterol: -0-
Saturated Fat: less than 1 gm
Beta Carotene: 9,250 I.U.
Vitamin C: 26 mg

Spinach, Brown Rice and Cheese Casserole

2 10 oz. packages of frozen, chopped Spinach

2 cups cooked Brown Rice

1 10 3/4 oz. can of condensed

Cream of Mushroom Soup

1/4 cup grated Parmesan Cheese

1 teaspoon Onion Powder

Salt and Pepper to taste

Thaw spinach then toss with brown rice. Mix together soup and seasonings then mix well with spinach and brown rice. Place mixture in casserole dish sprayed with non-stick spray. Sprinkle cheese on top. Bake at 350 degrees for 35 minutes.

Number of Servings: 4
Nutritional Analysis Per Serving:
Calories: 217
Fat: 5 gm (20%)
Fiber: 3.5 gm
Cholesterol: 5 mg
Saturated Fat: 4 gm
Beta Carotene: 9,200 I.U.
Vitamin C: 20 mg

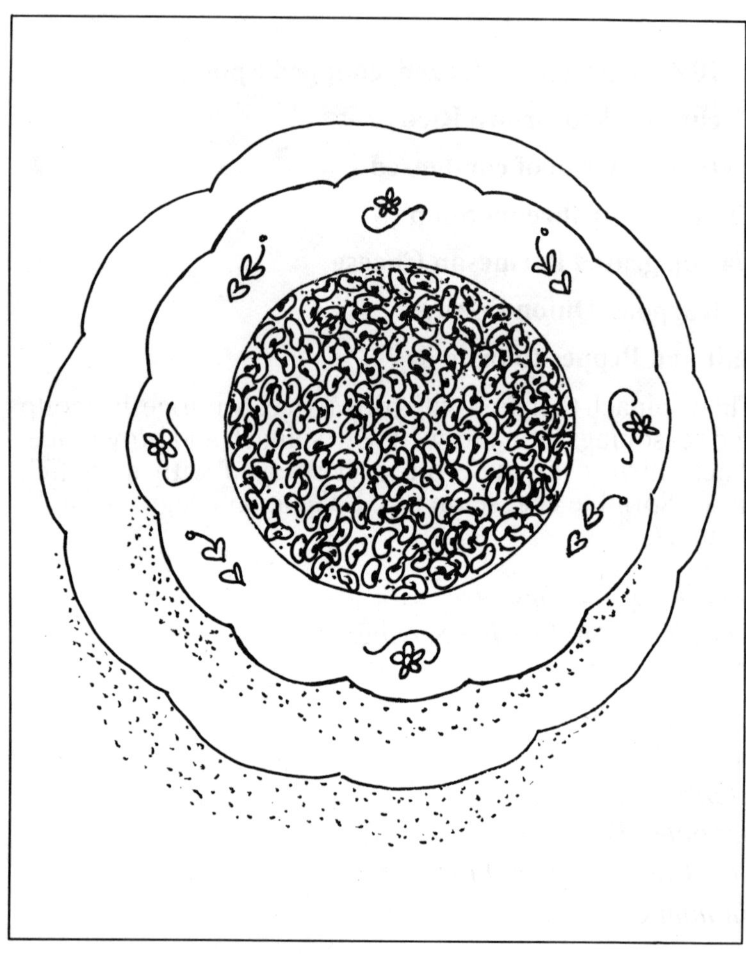

Hoppin' John

Hoppin' John

1 pound dried Black-Eyed Peas

1 teaspoon Cayenne Pepper

1 chopped Onion

1 cup raw Brown Rice

Salt and Pepper to taste

Put beans in 6 cups of water and boil for two minutes, cover, remove from heat and allow to sit for at least one hour. Return beans to a boil, add cayenne pepper, lower heat and allow to simmer for 45 minutes. Add onion, salt and pepper and allow to cook for another 45 minutes. Add raw brown rice and allow to cook for 45 minutes.

Number of Servings: 6
Nutritional Analysis Per Serving:
Calories: 250
Fat: 1 gm (4%)
Fiber: 1 gm
Cholesterol: -0-
Saturated Fat: less than 1 gm
Beta Carotene: 20 I.U.
Vitamin C: 3 mg

Shepherd's Pie

1 pound Potatoes
1/2 cup Skim Milk
1/2 cup Non-Fat Yogurt
Dash of Salt and Pepper
Filling:
1 tablespoon Olive Oil
1 chopped Onion
1 cube Chicken Bouillon
2 cups Low-Fat Cottage Cheese

Boil peeled, quartered potatoes in pot of water with a dash of salt until tender (15 - 20 minutes). While potatoes are boiling, in a skillet sauté onion in olive oil; when clear, set aside and allow to cool. When potatoes are finished cooking, drain through colander, mash well and allow to cool. Add milk, yogurt, salt and pepper to potatoes and mix completely.

Filling. Dissolve bouillon in 1 tablespoon of boiling water. Mix together onion, bouillon and cottage cheese.

Spray 9 to 10 inch casserole dish with non-stick spray. Spread half of potatoes, over bottom of casserole dish. Spread filling evenly over potatoes. Add second half of potatoes and spread evenly over filling. Bake in oven at 350 degrees for 30 minutes or until top is slightly browned.

Number of Servings: 4
Nutritional Analysis Per Serving:
Calories: 244
Fat: 4 gm (4%)
Fiber: 1 gm
Cholesterol: 6 mg
Saturated Fat: less than 1 gm
Beta Carotene: 85 I.U.
Vitamin C: 30 mg

Spinach and Cheese Pie

2 10 oz. packages of frozen, chopped Spinach

2 cups Low-Fat Cottage Cheese

2 sliced Leeks

1 teaspoon Olive Oil

Sprinkle with Parmesan Cheese
(no more than 1 tablespoon)

Salt and Pepper to Taste

Sauté leeks in olive oil until clear. Thaw and wash spinach in colander. Allow to drain thoroughly. In large mixing bowl, combine spinach with leeks, cottage cheese and salt and pepper. Spread into 9 or 10 inch casserole dish sprayed with non-stick spray. Sprinkle with Parmesan cheese. Bake at 350 degrees for 30 minutes.

Number of Servings: 4
Nutritional Analysis Per Serving:
Calories: 135
Fat: 4 gm (28%)
Fiber: 1 gm
Cholesterol: 5 mg
Saturated Fat: less than 1 gm
Beta Carotene: 10,000 I.U.
Vitamin C: 25 mg

Rotini and Broccoli Cheese Bake

1 bunch well chopped Broccoli
1 cup Low-Fat Cottage Cheese
1 cup Macaroni
6 toasted and cubed slices of Whole Wheat Bread
1/3 cup Skim Milk
2 thinly sliced Onions
2 pressed cloves of Garlic
1 tablespoon Olive Oil
Dash of Salt and Pepper
Parmesan Cheese (no more than 1 tablespoon)

Sauté onion and garlic in olive oil until clear. Add broccoli to skillet, cover and allow to simmer for 10 minutes on low heat. While broccoli is simmering, boil macaroni until *al dente,* approximately 8 minutes. In mixing bowl combine cottage cheese, skim milk, salt and pepper. When broccoli and macaroni are finished cooking, drain through colander then add to cheese mixture. Stir together well. Cover bottom of 9 or 10 inch casserole dish evenly with whole wheat cubes. Spoon in broccoli and cheese mixture. Sprinkle any remaining whole wheat cubes on top and garnish with Parmesan cheese.

Number of Servings: 6
Nutritional Analysis Per Serving:
Calories: 167
Fat: 4 gm (20%)
Fiber: 1 gm
Cholesterol: 2 mg
Saturated Fat: 1 gm
Beta Carotene: 1,200 I.U.
Vitamin C: 36 mg

Colorful Potato Casserole

6 thinly sliced Potatoes

3 grated Carrots

1 bunch diced Scallions

1 chopped Onion

1/3 cup Water

1 teaspoon of Oregano

Mix together all of the above ingredients except oregano. Put into 9 or 10 inch casserole dish sprayed with non-stick spray. Sprinkle with oregano. Cover and bake at 350 degrees for one hour.

Number of Servings: 6
Nutritional Analysis Per Serving:
Calories: 140
Fat: -0-
Fiber: 1 gm
Cholesterol: -0-
Saturated Fat: -0-
Beta Carotene: 10,375 I.U.
Vitamin C: 27 mg

Lentil and Brown Rice Loaf

2 cups cooked Lentils

1 cup cooked Brown Rice

1/2 cup diced Onion

3/4 cup seasoned Bread Crumbs

5 tablespoons Tomato Paste

1/2 cup of Water

Dash of Salt and Pepper

Mix all ingredients together in a large mixing bowl until well blended. Put into 9 or 10 inch casserole dish sprayed with non-stick spray. Bake at 350 degrees for 45 minutes. May be served with low-fat gravies and sauces.

Number of Servings: 4
Nutritional Analysis Per Serving:
Calories: 227
Fat: 1.5 gm (6%)
Fiber: 1 gm
Cholesterol: -0-
Saturated Fat: less than 1 gm
Beta Carotene: 1,000 I.U.
Vitamin C: 11 mg

Curried Lentils

4 cups cooked Lentils

2 15 oz. cans of Tomato Sauce

2 thinly sliced Carrots

1 diced Onion

1 pressed clove of Garlic

2 teaspoons Curry Powder

In medium size sauce pan bring tomato sauce, onion, garlic, curry powder and 1 cup of water to a simmer. Add lentils and carrots and allow to simmer for 20 to 30 minutes on low heat.

Number of Servings: 4
Nutritional Analysis Per Serving:
Calories: 300
Fat: 1 gm (3%)
Fiber: less than 1 gm
Cholesterol: -0-
Saturated Fat: -0-
Beta Carotene: 12,000 I.U.
Vitamin C: 40 mg

Bean Burgers

2 15 oz. cans of Pinto Beans

1 cup cooked Brown Rice

1/2 cup diced Onion

5 tablespoons Tomato Paste

Dash of Salt and Pepper

Sauté onion until clear. While onion is cooking, mash beans and brown rice together until well mixed. Add onion. Stir in tomato paste. Add salt and pepper to taste. Shape into patties and place on cookie sheet sprayed with non-stick spray. Bake in oven at 325 degrees for 30 minutes.

Number of Servings: 8
Nutritional Analysis Per Serving:
Calories: 153
Fat: less than 1 gm (4%)
Fiber: 5 gm
Cholesterol: -0-
Saturated Fat: -0-
Beta Carotene: 500 I.U.
Vitamin C: 5 mg

Lentil and Rice Burgers

1 cup cooked Lentils

1 chopped Onion

2 pressed cloves of Garlic

1 cup cooked Brown Rice

2 tablespoons Worcestershire Sauce

1 cup Corn Meal

Dash of Paprika

Dash of Salt and Pepper

In large bowl mix together all above ingredients well, except corn meal. Shape into patties. Pour corn meal into shallow dish. Coat both sides of each patty with corn meal. Place on cookie sheet sprayed with non-stick spray. Bake in a 350 degree oven for 30 - 40 minutes.

Number of Servings: 4
Nutritional Analysis Per Serving:
Calories: 152
Fat: less than 1 gm (4%)
Fiber: 2 gm
Cholesterol: -0-
Saturated Fat: -0-
Beta Carotene: 47 I.U.
Vitamin C: 4 mg

Vegetable Stir Fry

1 pound cut Green Beans

4 thinly sliced Carrots

1 head Broccoli

3 chopped stalks of Kale

3 pressed cloves of Garlic

1 teaspoon finely minced Ginger

1 teaspoon Olive Oil

1 tablespoon Soy Sauce

2 teaspoons Corn Starch

Make soy sauce gravy by combining 1/2 cup of water, soy sauce and corn starch in skillet over medium heat. Stir until all lumps have disappeared. In skillet sauté garlic and ginger in olive oil. Add cut green beans, carrots, broccoli, cut into flowerets, and kale. Add soy sauce mixture. Allow to simmer for 10 minutes; stir occasionally. This dish is especially good if served over rice.

Number of Servings: 6
Nutritional Analysis Per Serving:
Calories: 50
Fat: trace
Fiber: 1 gm
Cholesterol: -0-
Saturated Fat: -0-
Beta Carotene: 15,000 I.U.
Vitamin C: 55 mg

Risotto

1 1/2 cups long grain Rice

6 cubes Chicken Bouillon

2 chopped Shallots

1 tablespoon Olive Oil

1/4 cup Parmesan Cheese

1 cup Green Peas

Salt and Pepper to taste

Dissolve bouillon cubes in 4 cups of boiling water. In skillet sauté shallots in olive oil just until soft. Add rice to skillet. Stir frequently for one or two minutes then add 2 cups of broth. Allow rice to absorb three-quarters of the liquid then add the remaining broth. Allow rice to absorb most of liquid. Taste rice and test tenderness. If rice needs more liquid add additional broth. Add green peas three minutes before serving. The rice should be slightly moist when served. Remove from heat and stir in cheese. Salt and pepper to taste.

Number of Servings: 8
Nutritional Analysis Per Serving:
Calories: 185
Fat: 3 gm (16%)
Fiber: trace
Cholesterol: 3 mg
Saturated Fat: 1 gm
Beta Carotene: 155 I.U.
Vitamin C: 6 mg

Risotto with Seafood

1 1/2 cups long grain Rice
2 chopped Shallots
2 pressed cloves of Garlic
1 stalk of Celery, chopped
6 Shrimp, shelled and de-veined
6 well cleaned Clams (in shell)
6 well cleaned Mussels (in shell and de-bearded)
1 tablespoon Olive Oil
1/2 cup Dry White Wine
3 tablespoons Italian Seasonings
Salt and Pepper to taste

In large pot steam clams and mussels in 2 cups of water over medium heat until shells open slightly. Remove from pot as they open, draining liquid from shell over pot and place clams and mussels in bowl. Note: Discard any shells that do not open. Separate clams and mussels from their shells. Pour any excess liquid in bowl back into pot. In skillet, sauté shallots in olive oil until soft. Add garlic and celery and sauté until soft. Stir in clams, mussels and shrimp until shrimp are bright pink and clams and mussels are firm. Do not overcook - seafood will become rubbery. Remove seafood from skillet, set aside and keep warm. Pour rice into skillet. Add reserved seafood broth. Add wine and seasonings. Stir ingredients well, mixing thoroughly. Bring to a boil, lower heat and allow to simmer for 20 minutes or until rice is cooked but firm and most of the liquid has been absorbed. Remove from heat. Add seafood. Toss rice and seafood with fork. Salt and pepper to taste.

Number of Servings: 8
Nutritional Analysis Per Serving:
Calories: 210
Fat: 4 gm (19%)
Fiber: less than 1 gm
Cholesterol: 30 mg
Saturated Fat: less than 1 gm
Beta Carotene: 35 I.U.
Vitamin C: 4 mg

Paella Valenciana

1 boneless, skinless, cleaned Chicken Breast
2 cubes Chicken Bouillon
2 cups of medium grain Rice (Spanish, if possible)
3 pressed cloves of Garlic
1 chopped Onion
1 28 oz. can of Italian Plum Tomatoes
1 cup cut, cleaned Green Beans
1 cup frozen Peas
1 tablespoon Olive Oil
2 sprigs Rosemary
1 teaspoon Saffron
2 Lemons

Cut chicken breast into small strips. Brown in skillet on low heat in olive oil until very browned. While chicken is cooking, open can of tomatoes and carefully drain liquid into measuring cup. Dissolve bouillon in 1/4 cup very warm water. When chicken is finished cooking remove from heat. Check tomatoes to be sure no additional liquid has settled into the bottom of the container; if it has, pour liquid into measuring cup with other liquid. Place tomatoes only (no liquid) in skillet on low heat. Stir often using fork, mashing tomatoes while stirring to mix well with olive oil. While tomatoes are cooking measure liquid from tomatoes, chicken bouillon and add any additional warm water for a total of 3 cups of liquid. After tomatoes have been cooking for 20 minutes. Add garlic and onion then sauté for another 15 minutes. Add rice and slowly add 4 cups of liquid. Once rice and liquid have settled add saffron. Cook on low heat for 15 minutes, then add chicken, green beans, peas and rosemary. Allow to cook for an additional 15 minutes. Check rice to be sure it is fully cooked. Remove from heat. Allow to set for five minutes. Serve warm with lemon wedges.

Number of Servings: 8
Nutritional Analysis Per Serving:
Calories: 257
Fat: 3 gm (10%)
Fiber: 4 gm
Cholesterol: 10 mg
Saturated Fat: less than 1 gm
Beta Carotene: 1,000 I.U.
Vitamin C: 28 mg

Breaded Chicken

4 boneless, skinless, cleaned Chicken Breasts

1 cup of Skim Milk

1 Egg White

2 cups seasoned Bread Crumbs

1 tablespoon Italian Seasonings

1 tablespoon Olive Oil

Salt and Pepper to taste

Pour milk into bowl, add egg white and whisk with fork. Place chicken in bowl and allow to soak. Pour bread crumbs, seasonings, salt and pepper into brown paper bag; shake well. While olive oil is warming in skillet, shake each chicken breast in bag individually and place on plate. After all breasts have been breaded, carefully place in skillet. Allow to cook on each side for 10 minutes over medium heat. Do not turn too often as breading will fall off easily.

Number of Servings: 4
Nutritional Analysis Per Serving:
Calories: 254
Fat: 7 gm (26%)
Fiber: -0-
Cholesterol: 74 mg
Saturated Fat: 2 gm
Beta Carotene: 145 I.U.
Vitamin C: trace

Stuffed Chicken Breasts

4 boneless, skinless, cleaned Chicken Breasts

2 cups Bread Crumbs

1 finely chopped Onion

1 tablespoon Italian Seasonings

1 tablespoon Olive Oil

Salt and Pepper to taste

Toothpicks

Sauté oil and onion in skillet until soft. In bowl combine bread crumbs and seasonings, mix well. Add oil, onion, 1/3 cup of warm water to the bread crumbs. Stir well. Place one large spoon full of the stuffing in the middle of each chicken breast. Roll each chicken breast with stuffing in center and skewer with three toothpicks to keep closed. Place chicken breasts in casserole dish with seam down. Cover with either lid or aluminum foil. Place any left over stuffing in casserole dish, sprinkle with warm water, cover and place in 350 degree oven with chicken for 30 - 40 minutes.

Number of Servings: 4
Nutritional Analysis Per Serving:
Calories: 243
Fat: 7.5 gm (27%)
Fiber: less than 1 gm
Cholesterol: 73 mg
Saturated Fat: 2 gm
Beta Carotene: 20 I.U.
Vitamin C: 3 mg

Rosemary Chicken

4 boneless, skinned, cleaned Chicken Breasts

2 cubes Chicken Bouillon

3 sprigs Rosemary

1 tablespoon Olive Oil

Cook chicken breasts on low heat, 10 minutes on each side, in olive oil. While chicken is cooking dissolve bouillon cubes in 1/2 cup of hot water. When chicken is finished cooking, add broth and rosemary to skillet with chicken. Cover and simmer for 10-15 minutes.

Number of Servings: 4
Nutritional Analysis Per Serving:
Calories: 173
Fat: 7 gm (35%)
Fiber: -0-
Cholesterol: 73 mg
Saturated Fat: 1.5 gm
Beta Carotene: 20 I.U.
Vitamin C: -0-

Curried Chicken

4 boneless, skinned, cleaned Chicken Breasts

1/4 cup Honey

1 tablespoon Curry Powder

1/2 finely chopped Onion

1 pressed clove of Garlic

3 tablespoons Water

In a small saucepan combine all ingredients except chicken, stir well and simmer for 5 minutes on low heat. Place chicken breasts in a shallow baking dish. Pour curry sauce over chicken, cover dish and bake in 375 degree oven for 1 hour. Serve over rice or pasta.

Number of Servings: 4
Nutritional Analysis Per Serving:
Calories: 212
Fat: 3 gm (13%)
Fiber: -0-
Cholesterol: 73 mg
Saturated Fat: 1 gm
Beta Carotene: 20 I.U.
Vitamin C: 2 mg

Lemon Chicken

4 boneless, skinned, cleaned Chicken Breasts

2 Lemons

Grate lemon rind and set aside in bowl. Squeeze the juice from the lemon into another bowl. Place chicken breasts on plate and puncture with fork. Put a little bit of lemon rind in the center of each breast. Pour juice over breasts. Roll-up each breast, skewer with 3 toothpicks and place, seam side down, in casserole dish. Cover and bake at 350 degrees for 1 hour.

Number of Servings: 4
Nutritional Analysis Per Serving:
Calories: 150
Fat: 3 gm (18%)
Fiber: -0-
Cholesterol: 73 mg
Saturated Fat: 1 gm
Beta Carotene: 30 I.U.
Vitamin C: 15 mg

Turkey Pasties

1 cleaned, skinned, fully cooked Turkey Breast

2 peeled, cubed, cooked Potatoes

2 cubes Chicken Bouillon

2 teaspoons Corn Starch

2 teaspoons Poultry Seasoning

Pastry ingredients:

2 cups all-purpose Flour

1 teaspoon Salt

1/4 cup Vegetable Oil

3 tablespoons Skim Milk

Cut turkey into small strips. Dissolve bouillon in 1/2 cup hot water. Dissolve corn starch in 1 cup hot water. In skillet, heat broth until gently boiling. Add corn starch mixture slowly until broth becomes thick. If more cornstarch mixture is needed add slowly and sparingly. When finished set aside. In mixing bowl combine turkey, potatoes, gravy and poultry seasoning. Stir well and cover.

To prepare pastry:

Mix together in bowl flour and salt, stir together. Pour in oil and milk. Stir with pastry blender or fork. When well mixed separate into 2 balls. Cut each ball into two sections. Roll out each section on a piece of wax paper, be careful to make sure each section is rolled evenly and is at least 6 inches in diameter. When finished leave pastry on wax

(Continued on the next page)

paper and stack each section on top of the other; cover top piece with wax paper to prevent pastry from drying out.

Cut pre-prepared pastry in circles, approximately 6 inches in diameter or the size of a round serving bowl. Spoon pastie filling into center of each circle. Fold over into semicircle shape and seal with fork. When finished, place pasties on cookie sheet sprayed with non-stick spray and bake in 400 degree oven for 10-15 minutes or until lightly browned.

Number of Servings: 8
Nutritional Analysis Per Serving:
Calories: 232
Fat: 8 gm (31%)
Fiber: less than 1 gm
Cholesterol: 15 mg
Saturated Fat: less than 1 gm
Beta Carotene: 11 I.U.
Vitamin C: 5 mg

Pierogi

Cheese filling ingredients:

1 7.5 oz. Farmer's Cheese

1 Egg White

1 teaspoon Sugar

Chives or Green Onions to taste

Salt and Pepper to taste

Potato filling ingredients:

4 cooked, mashed Potatoes

3 tablespoons Skim Milk

Salt and Pepper to taste

Dough ingredients:

3 cups all-purpose Flour

1 cup Potato Filling

1 Egg White

1 cup Potato Water
(water used to boil potatoes for filling)

Dash of Salt

To prepare fillings:

Mix each set of ingredients and store in refrigerator in separate air-tight containers. Note: Any left over filling may be frozen until ready to use.

(Continued on the next page)

To prepare dough:

Mix together flour, potato filling, egg white and salt. Add just enough water to hold dough together. Roll into ball. Cut ball into two sections. Cut each section into three or four more sections. Roll out very thin using rolling pin or pasta machine (do not use noodle cutting mechanism). Cut rolled dough into circles using drinking glass. Spoon one type of each filling into the center of each circle. Fold dough over filling and seal with fork. Drop each pierogi into pot of boiling water and allow to boil until pierogi floats to the top (do not put more than six into pot at one time). Remove from pot, drain in colander, then place on plate to cool. When cool, put in air-tight container and store in either freezer or refrigerator. When ready to serve sauté pierogi in skillet with non-stick spray until lightly browned.

Number of Servings: 12
Nutritional Analysis Per Serving:
Calories: 158
Fat: trace (2%)
Fiber: less than 1 gm
Cholesterol: 1 mg
Saturated Fat: less than 1 gm
Beta Carotene: 136 I.U.
Vitamin C: 10 mg

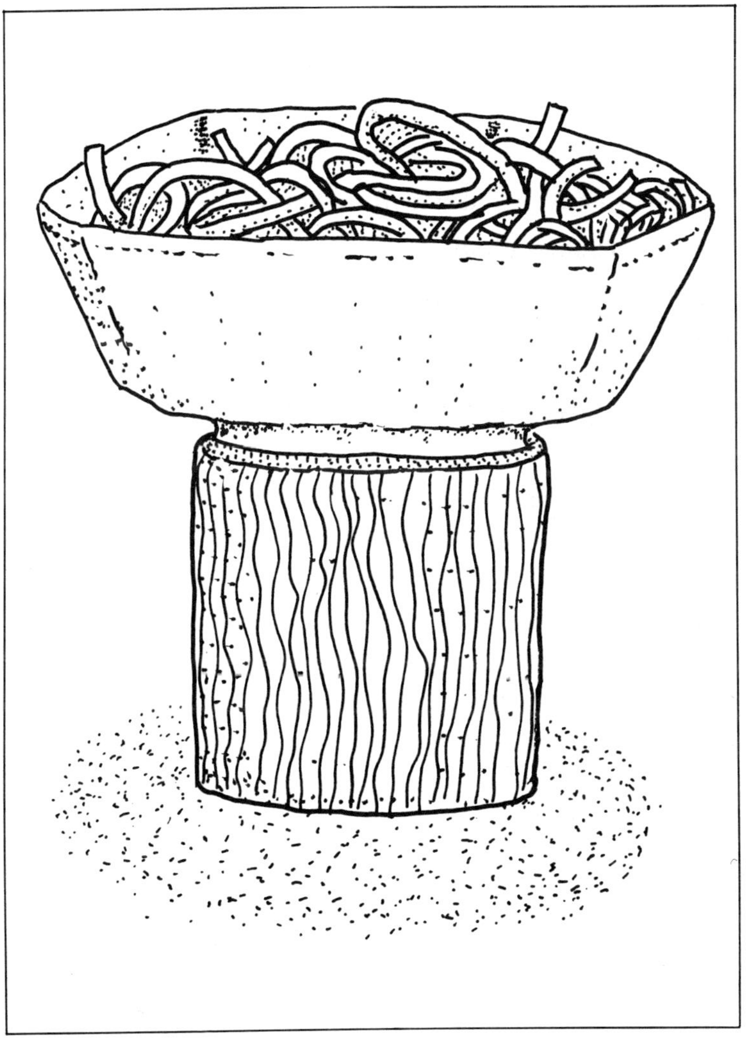

Fettuccine

Fettuccine with Ricotta Cheese

1 package of Fettuccine Noodles

1 teaspoon Olive Oil

1 chopped Leek

2 cups Reduced-Fat Ricotta Cheese

1/4 cup crushed Basil

Parmesan Cheese to taste (no more than 1 tablespoon)

Prepare noodles. Drain through colander. Pour hot noodles into bowl. Toss with olive oil. Add ricotta cheese and toss well. Sprinkle with basil and serve. Sprinkle with Parmesan cheese.

Number of Servings: 8
Nutritional Analysis Per Serving:
Calories: 261
Fat: 4 gm (13%)
Fiber: -0-
Cholesterol: 57 mg
Saturated Fat: less than 1 gm
Beta Carotene: 13 I.U.
Vitamin C: 16 mg

Fettuccine with Tomatoes

1 package of Fettuccine Noodles

1 pound Tomatoes

1 tablespoon Olive Oil

2 pressed cloves of Garlic

1/4 cup crushed Basil

Wash and cut tomatoes into wedges (discard the seeds). In a skillet slowly heat olive oil. When slightly warm, add garlic. After a minute or so add tomatoes. Cook for 3 or 4 minutes, then cover and set aside. Cook fettuccine until *al dente,* drain then add to tomato mixture in skillet. Add basil. Stir and cook over medium heat for one minute.

Number of Servings: 8
Nutritional Analysis Per Serving:
Calories: 241
Fat: 5 gm (17%)
Fiber: less than 1 gm
Cholesterol: 55 mg
Saturated Fat: less than 1 gm
Beta Carotene: 347 I.U.
Vitamin C: 11 mg

Pasta and Beans

2 15 oz. cans of Navy Beans
1 8 oz. package of short Pasta
1 28 oz. can of Plum Tomatoes
3 cubes Chicken Bouillon
1 tablespoon Olive Oil
1 sliced Onion
2 pressed cloves of Garlic
1 stalk of Celery, chopped
2 peeled, sliced Carrots
3 tablespoons chopped Parsley
Dash of Salt and Pepper

In soup pot sauté olive oil, onion and garlic. After a couple of minutes add celery and carrots. Add beans, 8 cups of water and bouillon cubes. Cover and cook over medium heat for 45 minutes to an hour. Cut tomatoes into small pieces and add to pot. Add parsley, salt and pepper. Cook over medium heat until beans are tender, 2 to 3 hours. When beans are tender, remove from heat. Carefully use potato masher and mash beans until mixture is thick but do not mash more than half of the beans. Return to heat. Add pasta and cook 5 minutes. Remove from heat and allow to set for 5 minutes. Serve with french bread and Parmesan cheese.

Number of Servings: 12
Nutritional Analysis Per Serving:
Calories: 150
Fat: 2 gm (12%)
Fiber: 4 gm
Cholesterol: trace
Saturated Fat: less than 1 gm
Beta Carotene: 3,916 I.U.
Vitamin C: 13 mg

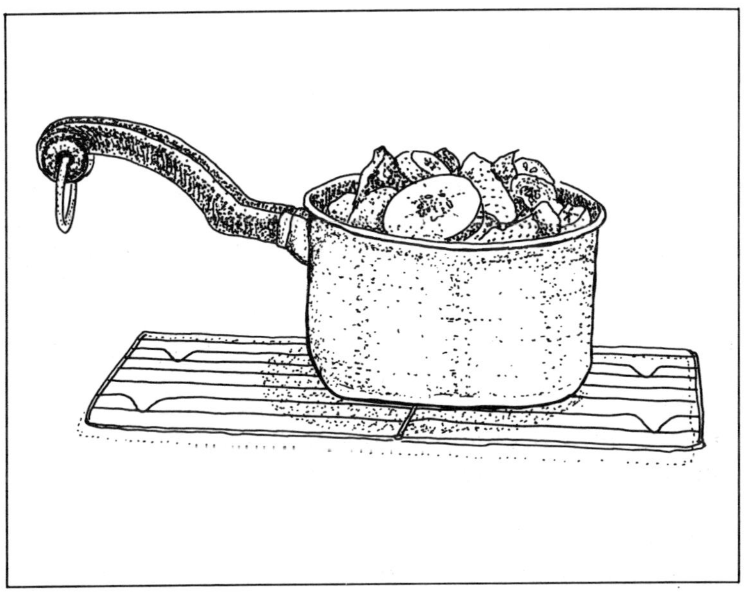

Ratatouille

Ratatouille

2 unpeeled, cubed Eggplants
3 pounds ripe, peeled chopped Tomatoes
1 pound chopped Zucchini
2 coarsely chopped Onions
1 Green Pepper, seeded and cut into strips
1 Red Pepper, seeded and cut into strips
1 teaspoon Olive Oil
4 pressed cloves of Garlic
1 teaspoon Thyme
1 teaspoon Basil
1 teaspoon Oregano
Salt and Pepper to taste

Place eggplant in colander, sprinkle with salt and drain for 20 minutes. In a large skillet sauté onions, peppers, and garlic in olive oil. When onions become clear add tomatoes and cook on low heat for five minutes. Remove mixture from skillet and put in covered bowl. Return skillet to heat. Sauté zucchini for 5 - 10 minutes. Add zucchini to bowl of other vegetables and cover. Pat eggplant dry with paper towel. Put in skillet and sauté for 10 minutes. Add previously sautéed vegetables from bowl to skillet. Heat mixture together with thyme, basil, oregano, salt and pepper for 45 minutes over medium heat.

Number of Servings: 8
Nutritional Analysis Per Serving:
Calories: 75
Fat: less than 1 gm (9%)
Fiber: 4 gm
Cholesterol: -0-
Saturated Fat: -0-
Beta Carotene: 2,000 I.U.
Vitamin C: 67 mg

Superb Spaghetti Sauce

3 ripe, whole Tomatoes

2 15 oz. cans of Tomato Sauce

1 6 oz. can of Tomato Paste

1 15 oz. can of Garbanzo Beans

2 thinly sliced Leeks

2 pressed cloves of Garlic

1 teaspoons Olive Oil

1 tablespoon chopped Parsley

1 tablespoon chopped Oregano

In skillet sauté leeks and garlic in olive oil. While these are cooking cut tomatoes into medium size pieces. Add tomato sauce and tomato paste to skillet and stir well until all ingredients are well combined. While ingredients are simmering on low heat. Mash garbanzo beans in juice with potato masher. Add to skillet and mix well. Add parsley and oregano. Cook for 15 - 20 minutes or until mixture is thick and hot. Serve over spaghetti.

Number of Servings: 8
Nutritional Analysis Per Serving:
Calories: 125
Fat: 2 gm (12%)
Fiber: 4 gm
Cholesterol: -0-
Saturated Fat: less than 1 gm
Beta Carotene: 1,697 I.U.
Vitamin C: 33 mg

Turkey Meatballs

1 pound Ground Turkey Breast

1 finely chopped Onion

2 pressed cloves of Garlic

1 teaspoon Olive Oil

1 tablespoon Rosemary

1 Egg White

In skillet sauté onion and garlic in olive oil until onion is clear. Set aside and allow to cool. In bowl combine turkey and egg white. Mix until well combined. Sprinkle rosemary over turkey; mix in. Add onion, garlic and olive oil to turkey and mix well. Do not clean skillet. Form turkey into small balls. Place meatballs in skillet, turning often, simmer on low heat for 30 minutes or until browned evenly and thoroughly cooked.

Number of Servings: 4
Nutritional Analysis Per Serving:
Calories: 207
Fat: 5 gm (22%)
Fiber: less than 1 gm
Cholesterol: 78 mg
Saturated Fat: 1 gm
Beta Carotene: -0-
Vitamin C: 3 mg

Spaghetti Carbonara

1 package of Spaghetti

1 tablespoon Olive Oil

2 Egg Whites

1/4 cup grated Parmesan Cheese

2 tablespoons Imitation Bacon (textured vegetable protein)

1 tablespoon Basil

1 tablespoon Oregano

Salt and Pepper to taste

Cook and drain spaghetti. Put directly into large bowl. Add egg whites, olive oil and toss well. Add Parmesan cheese and toss well. Place onto serving dishes and sprinkle with bacon, basil, oregano, salt and pepper.

Number of Servings: 6
Nutritional Analysis Per Serving:
Calories: 160
Fat: 5 gm (27%)
Fiber: less than 1 gm
Cholesterol: 3 mg
Saturated Fat: 1 gm
Beta Carotene: 29 I.U.
Vitamin C: -0-

Spaghetti and Squid

1 package of Spaghetti Noodles

1/2 pound small pieces Squid, cleaned

2 tablespoons finely chopped Onion

1 pressed clove of Garlic

1 teaspoon Olive Oil

1 28 oz. can of Plum Tomatoes

1/2 cup White Wine

Sauté onion and garlic in olive oil until onion is clear. Add tomatoes and cook over medium heat for 15 minutes. Add squid and cook for an additional 10 minutes on low heat. Add wine. Cover skillet and simmer for 50 - 60 minutes, stirring occasionally. When finished, leave covered and set aside. Cook pasta and drain. Spoon sauce over noodles on individual plates.

Number of Servings: 6
Nutritional Analysis Per Serving:
Calories: 216
Fat: 2 gm (1%)
Fiber: less than 1 gm
Cholesterol: 19 mg
Saturated Fat: less than 1 gm
Beta Carotene: 2,000 I.U.
Vitamin C: 20 mg

Spaghetti with Veggies

1 package of Spaghetti

2 cups thinly sliced Carrots

2 cups Broccoli Flowerets

1 tablespoon Olive Oil

1/4 cup Parmesan Cheese

In large pot, cook spaghetti. While spaghetti is cooking, warm olive oil on low heat. Add carrots and broccoli. Sauté for 10 minutes stirring often. When spaghetti is finished cooking and drained, toss with Parmesan cheese. Add carrots and broccoli to pasta, then toss.

Number of Servings: 6
Nutritional Analysis Per Serving:
Calories: 172
Fat: 4 gm (22%)
Fiber: 1 gm
Cholesterol: 3 mg
Saturated Fat: 1 gm
Beta Carotene: 10,000 I.U.
Vitamin C: 34 mg

Linguine with Peppers

1 package of Linguine

2 Red Peppers, cored and cut into strips

2 Green Peppers, cored and cut into strips

1 28 oz. can of Plum Tomatoes

1 tablespoon Olive Oil

2 pressed cloves of Garlic

1 finely chopped Onion

1 tablespoon Oregano

Parmesan Cheese to taste (no more than 1 tablespoon)

In skillet, sauté garlic and onion in olive oil until soft. Add tomatoes and oregano. Mash with fork while stirring often. After ten minutes add red and green peppers. Allow to simmer on low heat in skillet for 20 - 30 minutes. Ten minutes before sauce is finished add linguine to boiling water and cook until *al dente.*

Number of Servings: 8
Nutritional Analysis Per Serving:
Calories: 297
Fat: 4 gm (11%)
Fiber: 1 gm
Cholesterol: 55 mg
Saturated Fat: less than 1 gm
Beta Carotene: 2,600 I.U.
Vitamin C: 76 mg

Macaroni and Snow Peas

1 package of short Macaroni

1/4 pound Snow Peas

1 pressed clove of Garlic

1 thinly sliced Onion

1 teaspoon Olive Oil

Sauté garlic and onion in olive oil on low heat until clear. Snip ends off snow peas and add to skillet. Cook macaroni, drain then toss with peas and seasonings. Salt and pepper to taste. Serve as a soup by allowing water to cook down and become thick.

Number of Servings: 8
Nutritional Analysis Per Serving:
Calories: 93
Fat: 2 gm (17%)
Fiber: 2 gm
Cholesterol: -0-
Saturated Fat: less than 1 gm
Beta Carotene: 52 I.U.
Vitamin C: 6 mg

Rotini and Pumpkin

1 package of Rotini

1 16 oz. can of Pumpkin

1 tablespoon Olive Oil

1 cup Salsa

Salt and Pepper to taste

Warm olive oil in skillet on low heat. Add pumpkin and cook for 20 minutes stirring constantly. Cover and remove from heat. Cook pasta and drain. Pour into large bowl. Add pumpkin and stir well. Salt and pepper to taste. Place onto individual serving dishes, spoon salsa on top.

Number of Servings: 8
Nutritional Analysis Per Serving:
Calories: 250
Fat: 3 gm (10%)
Fiber: 2 gm
Cholesterol: -0-
Saturated Fat: less than 1 gm
Beta Carotene: 13,680 I.U.
Vitamin C: 3 mg

Rotini and Broccoli Flowerets

1 package of Rotini

1 pound Broccoli Flowerets

1 cup No-Oil Herb Dressing

1 tablespoon Olive Oil

1 thinly sliced Onion

2 sliced Lemons

While broccoli is boiling, cook and drain rotini. Sauté onion in olive oil on low heat until soft; add broccoli. Cook for 15 minutes. Pour cooked rotini into large bowl, add broccoli and stir. Add dressing and mix well. Squeeze lemon juice over pasta and broccoli.

Number of Servings: 8
Nutritional Analysis Per Serving:
Calories: 254
Fat: 3 gm (10%)
Fiber: 2 gm
Cholesterol: -0-
Saturated Fat: less than 1 gm
Beta Carotene: 550 I.U.
Vitamin C: 33 mg

Rotini with Peas and Carrots

1 package of Rotini

1/2 pound shelled Peas

8 peeled, thinly sliced Carrots

1 tablespoon Olive Oil

1 tablespoon Parsley

2 tablespoons Parmesan Cheese

In large sauce pan boil 3 cups of water. Add carrots and peas. Cook for 10 minutes. At the same time cook rotini and drain. Pour rotini into large bowl, add carrots, peas, olive oil and Parmesan cheese. Toss well. Sprinkle with parsley.

Number of Servings: 8
Nutritional Analysis Per Serving:
Calories: 270
Fat: 3 gm (11%)
Fiber: 2 gm
Cholesterol: 2 mg
Saturated Fat: less than 1 gm
Beta Carotene: 20,000 I.U.
Vitamin C: 16 mg

Rotini and Spinach

1 package of Rotini

1 pound washed Spinach

1 cup Low-Fat Vinaigrette Dressing

Cook and drain rotini. While rotini is cooking, wash and drain spinach. In another large pot boil 3 cups of water and add spinach. Cook for 5 minutes, stirring frequently. Drain pasta and spinach separately. Pour rotini into large bowl, add spinach and vinaigrette and stir well.

Number of Servings: 10
Nutritional Analysis Per Serving:
Calories: 184
Fat: less than 1 gm (4%)
Fiber: 2 gm
Cholesterol: -0-
Saturated Fat: less than 1 gm
Beta Carotene: 2,948 I.U.
Vitamin C: 3 mg

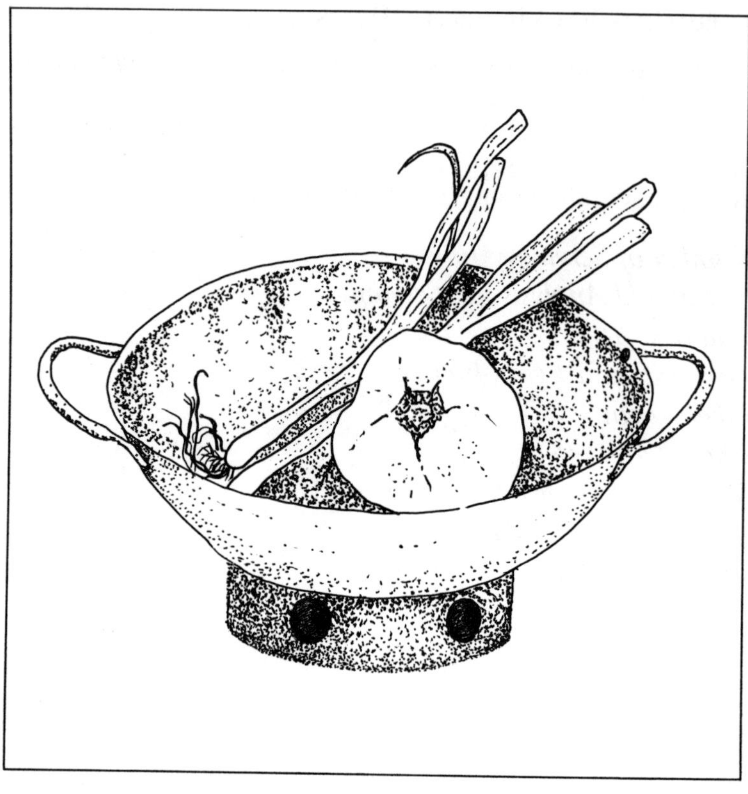

Vegetables, Herbs & Pasta

Vegetables, Herbs and Pasta

1 16 oz. package of Pasta

3 pounds of the following Vegetables in any combination:

carrots, broccoli, spinach, celery and onion

1 teaspoon each of the following Herbs:

salt, pepper, garlic powder, parsley

2 tablespoons Olive Oil

1 tablespoon Soy Sauce

Cook and drain pasta. Finely chop vegetables and sauté in olive oil. Add 1/2 cup of water and continue to cook for 10 minutes. Add herbs and soy sauce. Cook an additional 5 minutes. If needed, thicken with a small amount of corn starch. In a large bowl combine pasta and vegetable sauté.

Number of Servings: 10
Nutritional Analysis Per Serving:
Calories: 146
Fat: 3 gm (16%)
Fiber: 3 gm
Cholesterol: -0-
Saturated Fat: less than 1 gm
Beta Carotene: 9,500 I.U.
Vitamin C: 27 mg

Rice, Chicken and Spinach Casserole

3 cups cooked Brown Rice

1 pound cooked Spinach

2 boneless, skinless, cleaned Chicken Breasts

1 tablespoon Olive Oil

2 pressed cloves of Garlic

1 finely chopped Onion

2 cubes Chicken Bouillon

In skillet sauté chicken breasts in olive oil, garlic and onion. Dissolve bouillon in 2 cups of hot water. When chicken is well browned, remove from skillet and cut chicken into small strips. In a baking dish, sprayed with non-stick spray, spread one layer of rice on bottom, add bed of spinach, a few strips of chicken and 1/2 cup of broth. Then repeat again in same order. Bake for 35 minutes in preheated 350 degree oven.

Number of Servings: 8
Nutritional Analysis Per Serving:
Calories: 166
Fat: 3 gm (17%)
Fiber: 3 gm
Cholesterol: 24 mg
Saturated Fat: less than 1 gm
Beta Carotene: 4,000 I.U.
Vitamin C: 5 mg

Black Beans and Rice

1 cup cooked Black Beans

1 cup cooked long grain Rice

1 chopped Onion

2 pressed cloves of Garlic

2 tablespoons Hot Sauce

Salt and Pepper to taste

Sauté onion and garlic in olive oil until clear. Add onion, garlic and cooked rice to pot of cooked beans and remaining liquid. Add enough hot water to ensure that there are 3 cups of liquid in the pot. Add hot sauce, cover and cook for 30 - 45 minutes. Be careful to check liquid frequently and replenish if necessary.

Number of Servings: 4
Nutritional Analysis Per Serving:
Calories: 126
Fat: less than 1 gm (2%)
Fiber: 4 gm
Cholesterol: -0-
Saturated Fat: less than 1 gm
Beta Carotene: -0-
Vitamin C: 3 mg

Cauliflower and Rice Bake

1 pound Cauliflower

1 cup medium grain Rice

1 finely chopped Onion

2 cups Skim Milk

1 cup Bread Crumbs

Salt and Pepper to taste

Chop cauliflower into flowerets, boil for ten minutes in soup pot, drain and set aside. Bring two cups of water to a boil and add rice. Bring to a boil again, cover and cook for 15 minutes or until liquid is absorbed. While rice is boiling, sauté onion in skillet sprayed with non-stick spray until clear. Add cooked and drained rice to onion, stir well and allow to cook on low heat for 5 minutes. Pour rice into bowl, add skim milk, salt and pepper. Spray casserole dish with non-stick spray and sprinkle with bread crumbs. Add a layer of rice, then a layer of cauliflower, then a layer of bread crumbs. Repeat until all ingredients are in casserole dish. Top with bread crumbs. Bake uncovered in a preheated oven at 350 degrees for 30 - 40 minutes.

Number of Servings: 4
Nutritional Analysis Per Serving:
Calories: 268
Fat: less than 1 gm (2%)
Fiber: 2 gm
Cholesterol: 2 mg
Saturated Fat: less than 1 gm
Beta Carotene: 250 I.U.
Vitamin C: 40 mg

Rice and Lentils

1 cup long grain Rice

1/2 cup dry (red, if possible) Lentils

1 chopped Onions

3 pressed cloves of Garlic

4 cubes Chicken Bouillon

1 teaspoon Turmeric

1/2 teaspoon Cinnamon

Salt and Pepper to taste

Sauté onion until soft in skillet sprayed with non-stick spray. Add garlic and sauté briefly. Set onion and garlic aside. Put rice, lentils, turmeric and cinnamon in skillet and stir until well blended. While these ingredients are cooking in skillet dissolve bouillon cubes in 3 cups of water. Add broth to skillet as soon as possible, as well as onion and garlic. Cover and allow to simmer over medium heat for 40 - 45 minutes, stirring frequently, or until all of the liquid has been absorbed. Salt and pepper to taste just before serving.

Number of Servings: 4
Nutritional Analysis Per Serving:
Calories: 215
Fat: 1 gm (4%)
Fiber: 3 gm
Cholesterol: -0-
Saturated Fat: less than 1 gm
Beta Carotene: 5 I.U.
Vitamin C: 3 mg

Rice and Peas

2 cups long grain Rice

1 small package of frozen Green Peas

5 finely chopped Scallions

3 pressed cloves of Garlic

4 cubes Chicken Bouillon

1 tablespoon Olive Oil

3 tablespoons Parmesan Cheese

Sauté scallions until soft in skillet with olive oil. Add garlic and sauté briefly. Add rice and stir until well blended. While these ingredients are cooking in skillet dissolve bouillon cubes in 3 cups of water. Add to skillet as soon as possible. Cover and allow to simmer over medium heat for 15 minutes. Add peas and stir well. Continue to cook until all of the liquid has been absorbed. Serve portions sprinkled with Parmesan cheese.

Number of Servings: 6
Nutritional Analysis Per Serving:
Calories: 313
Fat: 4 gm (11%)
Fiber: 3 gm
Cholesterol: 3 mg
Saturated Fat: 1 gm
Beta Carotene: 378 I.U.
Vitamin C: 27 mg

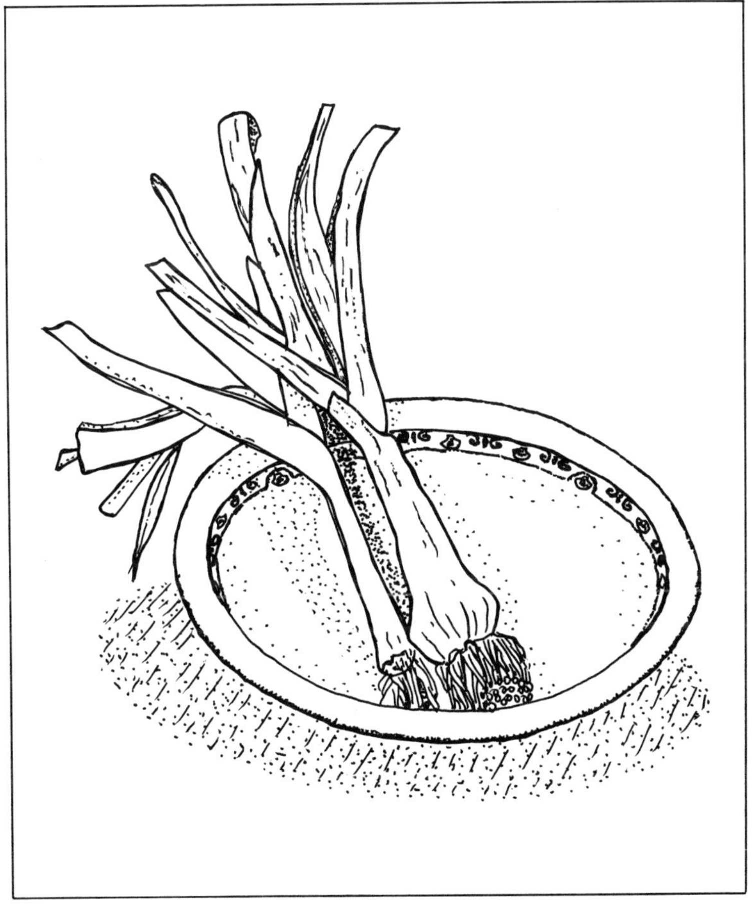

Leeks

Rice and Mixed Vegetables

2 cups long grain Rice

1 small package of frozen Mixed Vegetables

1 tablespoon Soy Sauce

Cook rice in covered sauce pan in four cups of water until water is almost completely absorbed. At the same time cook frozen vegetables over medium heat in separate pot. When rice and vegetables are completely cooked, put rice in large bowl, drain vegetables in colander and add to rice. Add soy sauce and mix very well.

Number of Servings: 6
Nutritional Analysis Per Serving:
Calories: 260
Fat: trace
Fiber: 1 gm
Cholesterol: -0-
Saturated Fat: -0-
Beta Carotene: 2,600 I.U.
Vitamin C: 3

FREE N' LEAN™ Cheese

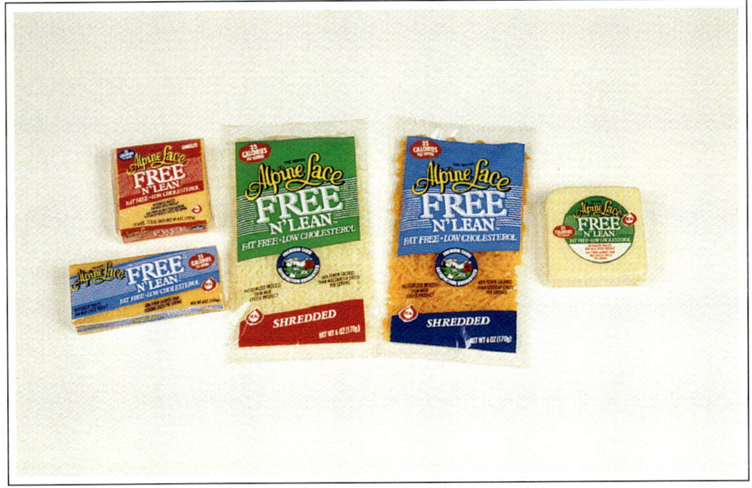

Cheese Fondue

2 cups shredded Alpine Lace® FREE N' LEAN™ American Cheese
1 cup Non-Fat Plain Yogurt
1 finely chopped Scallion
1 pressed clove of Garlic
1/2 cup dry White Wine
1 tablespoon Flour
Dash of Nutmeg

In a bowl toss cheese with flour and put aside. In a skillet sprayed with non-stick spray, sauté scallion and garlic on low heat until tender. Add wine to skillet and allow to simmer for 5 minutes. Add cheese a little at a time; stir until smooth and melted. While cheese is in skillet, drain yogurt through cheese cloth until most of the liquid has drained out. Remove skillet from heat, put in serving container, add yogurt and stir well. Dust with nutmeg before serving.

Number of Servings: 6
Nutritional Analysis Per Serving:
Calories: 120
Fat: -0-
Fiber: -0-
Cholesterol: -0-
Saturated Fat: -0-
Beta Carotene: 4 I.U.
Vitamin C: 1 mg

Cheese Soup

1 cup shredded Alpine Lace® FREE N' LEAN™ American Cheese
1/2 cup shredded Carrot
1/2 cup finely chopped Scallions
2 cups Skim Milk
3 cubes Chicken Bouillon
3 tablespoons Flour
Salt and Pepper to taste

In a large bowl mix together carrot and scallion. In a medium size saucepan, heat 2 cups of water with chicken bouillon cubes. Add carrot and scallion mixture. Allow mixture to boil then reduce heat. Cover and simmer until vegetables are soft. Add milk, flour, salt and pepper. Allow to cook on moderate heat until mixture thickens. Add cheese and stir until melted.

Number of Servings: 4
Nutritional Analysis Per Serving:
Calories: 134
Fat: less than 1 gm (3%)
Fiber: 1 gm
Cholesterol: 2 mg
Saturated Fat: less than 1 gm
Beta Carotene: 4,100 I.U.
Vitamin C: 4 mg

Macaroni and Cheese

2 cups Elbow Macaroni

2 cups cubed Alpine Lace® FREE N' LEAN™ American Cheese

2 cups Skim Milk

2 finely chopped Scallions

1 cup seasoned Bread Crumbs

1 tablespoon Flour

Dash of Salt and Pepper

In a bowl toss cheese with flour and set aside. In a skillet sprayed with non-stick spray, sauté scallion on low heat until tender. Add milk all at once and warm on low heat until simmering lightly. Add cheese and stir until melted. While making cheese mixture, cook macaroni according to package directions, drain and set aside. When macaroni is done and cheese is thoroughly melted, add cheese to bowl of macaroni and stir well. Turn into casserole dish, sprinkle with salt, pepper and bread crumbs. Bake in 350 degree oven for 20 minutes.

Number of Servings: 6
Nutritional Analysis Per Serving:
Calories: 205
Fat: less than 1 gm (2%)
Fiber: 1 gm
Cholesterol: 1 mg
Saturated Fat: less than 1 gm
Beta Carotene: 200 I.U.
Vitamin C: 2 mg

Pizza

2 - 3 cups all-purpose Flour

1 package of Active Dry Yeast

2 tablespoons Olive Oil

1/2 teaspoon Salt

1 15 oz. can of Pizza Sauce

1 teaspoon Basil

1 teaspoon Oregano

2 cups shredded Alpine Lace® FREE N' LEAN™ Mozzarella Cheese

2 cups shredded Alpine Lace® FREE N' LEAN™ Cheddar Cheese

1 diced Red Pepper

1 diced Green Pepper

1 chopped Onion

1 tablespoon Parmesan Cheese

1/2 cup cooked Mushrooms

To make crust, mix 1 1/2 cups of flour, yeast and salt. Add 1 cup warm water and oil. Stir together well. Using a spoon, mix in as much flour as possible. Form dough into ball then turn onto floured surface. Knead in remaining flour until dough is smooth and stiff, should be elastic. Try not to work dough for too long. Cover dough with warm dish cloth and allow to set for 10 - 15 minutes. Divide dough in half. Roll each half on lightly floured surface into a circle that will cover the bottom of the pizza pan. Transfer dough onto pizza pans sprayed with non-stick spray. Fold up edges of dough slightly. Pour pizza sauce on dough and spread with spoon until dough is well covered. Sprinkle with salt, pepper, basil and oregano. Cover with cheese, red pepper, green pepper, onion and mushrooms. Sprinkle with Parmesan cheese. Bake in 425 degree oven for 10 - 15 minutes or until cheese is lightly browned.

Number of Servings: 12
Nutritional Analysis Per Serving:
Calories: 210
Fat: 3 gm (12%)
Fiber: 1 gm
Cholesterol: -0-
Saturated Fat: less than 1 gm
Beta Carotene: 787 I.U.
Vitamin C: 26 mg

Veggie Sub-Sandwich

2 thinly sliced Carrots

1 thinly sliced stalk of Celery

1 thinly sliced Zucchini

1 thinly shopped Leek

2 tablespoons Low-Fat Vinaigrette Dressing

4 slices Alpine Lace® FREE N' LEAN™ Mozzarella Cheese

4 Sub-Sandwich Rolls

Sauté vegetables slowly in skillet sprayed with non-stick spray for 15 minutes. When finished spoon into rolls and top with Mozzarella cheese and dressing. Broil until cheese is melted.

Number of Servings: 4
Nutritional Analysis Per Serving:
Calories: 215
Fat: 2 gm (9%)
Fiber: 2 gm
Cholesterol: -0-
Saturated Fat: less than 1 gm
Beta Carotene: 10,200 I.U.
Vitamin C: 9 mg

Grilled Cheese Sandwich

8 slices Whole Wheat Bread

2 cups shredded Alpine Lace® FREE N' LEAN™ American Cheese

2 cups shredded Alpine Lace® FREE N' LEAN™ Mozzarella Cheese

Toppings:

Sliced Tomato, Chopped Green Pepper, Sliced Onion

Place two slices of bread in skillet sprayed with non-stick spray. Sprinkle bread liberally with mixture of both cheeses. Add two more slices of bread on top of cheese, add top slice of bread on cheese. Cook over low heat for five minutes. Check to see that cheese has begun to melt by lifting top slice of bread. If cheese is warm, carefully flip sandwiches so that other side can begin to brown. Bread will be lightly toasted and cheese soft when done. Top with vegetable slices, if desired.

Number of Servings: 4
Nutritional Analysis Per Serving:
Calories: 340
Fat: 2 gm (5%)
Fiber: 2 gm
Cholesterol: -0-
Saturated Fat: less than 1 gm
Beta Carotene: -0-
Vitamin C: -0-

Cheese Bean Burgers

1 15 oz. can of Pinto Beans

1 cup cooked Brown Rice

1/2 cup diced Onion

5 tablespoons Tomato Paste

1/2 cup small cubes of Alpine Lace® FREE N' LEAN™ American Cheese

4 slices of Alpine Lace® FREE N' LEAN™ American Cheese

Dash of Salt and Pepper

Sauté onion until clear. While onion is cooking, mash beans and brown rice together until well mixed. Add onion. Stir in tomato paste. Add salt and pepper to taste. Add cubes of cheese and mix well with bean and rice mixture until thoroughly combined. Shape into patties and place on cookie sheet sprayed with non-stick spray. Bake in oven at 325 degrees for 30 minutes.

Number of Servings: 6
Nutritional Analysis Per Serving:
Calories: 183
Fat: less than 1 gm (3%)
Fiber: 5 gm
Cholesterol: -0-
Saturated Fat: less than 1 gm
Beta Carotene: 337 I.U.
Vitamin C: 7 mg

Jalapeno Cheese Sauce

1 diced Jalapeno Pepper

2 cups shredded Alpine Lace® FREE N' LEAN™ American Cheese

1 cup Skim Milk

1 tablespoon Flour

Warm milk slowly in saucepan over low heat. Toss cheese with flour in bowl then add to milk in saucepan. Allow cheese and milk to simmer until mixture is completely smooth. When cheese is finished cooking, add jalapenos, mix well, then spoon cheese sauce over main dish.

Number of Servings: 4
Nutritional Analysis Per Serving:
Calories: 140
Fat: -0-
Fiber: -0-
Cholesterol: 1 mg
Saturated Fat: less than 1 gm
Beta Carotene: 212 I.U.
Vitamin C: trace

Bean Tacos

1 15 oz. can of Pinto or Kidney Beans
1 chopped Onion
1 tablespoon Chili Powder
2 teaspoons Olive Oil
1 box Taco Shells

Toppings:

Shredded Alpine Lace® FREE N' LEAN™ American Cheese
Non-Fat Yogurt
Chopped Tomato
Chopped Onion
Chopped Green Pepper
Shredded Lettuce
Hot Sauce

In small skillet sauté onion in oil until lightly browned. In mixing bowl combine onion, beans and chili powder. Mash beans with potato masher until thick in consistency. Spoon into taco shells and bake in 350 degree oven for 5 minutes. After removing from the oven, top with cheese, yogurt, tomato, onion, green pepper, lettuce and sauce.

Number of Servings: 8
Nutritional Analysis Per Serving:
Calories: 200
Fat: 3 gm (11%)
Fiber: 4 gm
Cholesterol: -0-
Saturated Fat: less than 1 gm
Beta Carotene: 364 I.U.
Vitamin C: 1 mg

Chicken Tacos

4 boneless, skinless, cleaned Chicken Breasts
2 pressed cloves of Garlic
1 teaspoon Ground Pepper
2 teaspoons Safflower Oil
1 box Taco Shells

Toppings:

Shredded Alpine Lace® FREE N' LEAN™ American Cheese
Non-Fat Yogurt
Chopped Tomato
Chopped Onion
Chopped Green Pepper
Shredded Lettuce
Hot Sauce

In skillet sauté garlic in oil. Add chicken and cook on low heat until lightly browned. When finished cut into thin strips while taco shells are warming in the oven. After removing shells from the oven, spoon in chicken, top with cheese, yogurt, tomato, onion, green pepper, lettuce and sauce.

Number of Servings: 8
Nutritional Analysis Per Serving:
Calories: 220
Fat: 4 gm (17%)
Fiber: 1 gm
Cholesterol: 48 mg
Saturated Fat: less than 1 gm
Beta Carotene: 377 I.U.
Vitamin C: 1 mg

Bean Enchiladas

1 15 oz. can of Pinto or Kidney Beans

1 chopped Onion

1 tablespoon Chili Powder

1 tablespoon Olive Oil

1 10 oz. can of Enchilada Sauce

1 cup grated Alpine Lace® FREE N' LEAN™ Mozzarella Cheese

8 Corn Tortillas

In medium size bowl, combine beans, onion, chili powder and oil. In skillet, mix 4 tablespoons of water and sauce. Heat until sauce is boiling. Place one tortilla in mixture and allow to simmer until tortilla is limp. Remove from skillet, allowing excess sauce to drip back into skillet, and place on plate. Spoon 1/2 cup of bean mixture onto tortilla and spread across center evenly. Roll up tortilla and set in 3" deep casserole pan with seam on the bottom. Make remaining tortillas and place them in pan in a single layer. Pour any remaining sauce over all tortillas. Sprinkle cheese on top. Cover and bake in preheated oven, 375 degrees, for 10 - 15 minutes. Uncover and continue to cook for 5 minutes, or until cheese is lightly browned.

Number of Servings: 8
Nutritional Analysis Per Serving:
Calories: 185
Fat: 3 gm (15%)
Fiber: 3 gm
Cholesterol: -0-
Saturated Fat: less than 1 gm
Beta Carotene: 261 I.U.
Vitamin C: 2 mg

Chicken Enchiladas

1/2 pound boneless, skinless, cooked Chicken Breast
1 chopped Onion
1 tablespoon Paprika
1 10 oz. can of Enchilada Sauce
1 cup grated Alpine Lace® FREE N' LEAN™ Mozzarella Cheese
8 Corn Tortillas

When chicken cools, cut into small, thin strips. In medium size bowl, combine chicken, onion, and paprika. In skillet, mix 4 tablespoons of water and sauce. Heat until sauce is boiling. Place one tortilla in mixture and allow to simmer until tortilla is limp. Remove from skillet, allowing excess sauce to drip back into skillet, and place on plate. Spoon 1/2 cup of chicken mixture onto tortilla and spread across center evenly. Roll up tortilla and set in 3" deep casserole pan, sprayed with non-stick spray, with seam on the bottom. Make remaining tortillas and place them in pan in a single layer. Pour any remaining sauce over all tortillas. Sprinkle cheese on top. Cover with foil and bake in preheated oven, 375 degrees, for 10 - 15 minutes. Remove foil and continue to cook for 5 minutes, or until cheese is lightly browned.

Number of Servings: 8
Nutritional Analysis Per Serving:
Calories: 151
Fat: 2 gm (13%)
Fiber: less than 1 gm
Cholesterol: 24 mg
Saturated Fat: less than 1 gm
Beta Carotene: 267 I.U.
Vitamin C: 2 mg

Parmesan Chicken

4 boneless, skinned, cleaned Chicken Breasts

2 cups Tomato Sauce

1 tablespoon Italian Seasoning

1 teaspoon Olive Oil

4 slices Alpine Lace® FREE N' LEAN™ Mozzarella Cheese

Salt and Pepper to taste

Parmesan Cheese to taste (no more than 1 tablespoon)

Cook chicken breasts on low heat, 5 minutes on each side, in olive oil. In cup mix Italian seasonings and tomato sauce together. Pour over cooking chicken and simmer for 10 - 15 minutes on low heat. When chicken is finished cooking place in casserole dish, with one slice of Mozzarella cheese on each chicken breast, put in 350 degree oven and bake until cheese is lightly browned. Remove from oven, place on serving dish and sprinkle with Parmesan cheese. Serve over a bed of rice or noodles.

Number of Servings: 4
Nutritional Analysis Per Serving:
Calories: 244
Fat: 6 gm (24%)
Fiber: -0-
Cholesterol: 73 mg
Saturated Fat: 1.5 gm
Beta Carotene: 1,213 I.U.
Vitamin C: 16 mg

Lasagna - Vegetarian Style

1 package of Lasagna Noodles

2 15 oz. cans of Tomato Sauce

2 small packages of frozen (defrosted), chopped Spinach

1 cup Reduced-Fat Farmer's Cheese

1 cup Low-Fat Cottage Cheese

6 oz. thinly sliced Alpine Lace® FREE N' LEAN™ Mozzarella Cheese

1 chopped Onion

2 teaspoons Basil

1 pressed clove of Garlic

1 tablespoon Olive Oil

In skillet, warm olive oil then sauté onion and garlic. Wash and drain spinach in colander. Pour spinach onto towel and dry. Add spinach to skillet and cook until soft; remove from heat. Put spinach into bowl. Add Farmer's cheese, cottage cheese, and basil, mix well. Place one layer of cooked noodles in 13x9x2 inch casserole dish sprayed with non-stick spray. Spoon spinach and cheese mixture onto noodles, cover evenly. Add layer of sliced Mozzarella cheese. Spoon on tomato sauce and spread evenly.

(Continued on the next page)

Continue to add layers until pan is full. Make sure noodles completely cover the top. Sprinkle noodles with Parmesan cheese. Cover and bake in 375 degree oven for 30 - 40 minutes.

Number of Servings: 12
Nutritional Analysis Per Serving:
Calories: 182
Fat: 2 gm (9%)
Fiber: less than 1 gm
Cholesterol: 2 mg
Saturated Fat: less than 1 gm
Beta Carotene: 2,500 I.U.
Vitamin C: 20 mg

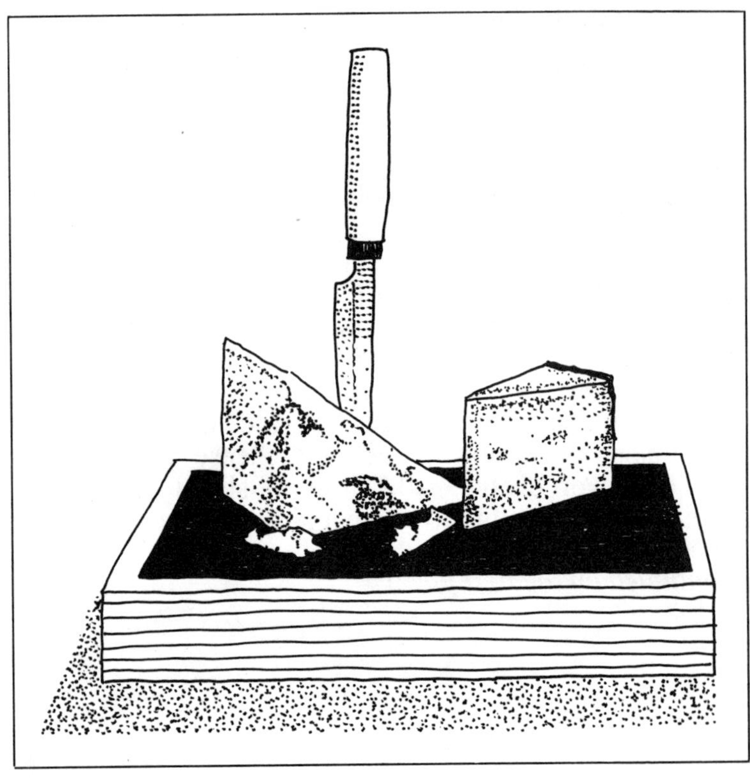

Eggplant Parmigiana

1 peeled, thinly sliced Eggplant

1 cup shredded Alpine Lace® FREE N' LEAN™ Cheddar Cheese

1/2 cup seasoned Bread Crumbs

1 Egg White

1 15 oz. can of Tomato Sauce

1 tablespoon Parmesan Cheese

Dip eggplant in egg white and make sure it is well covered. Pour bread crumbs into small brown paper bag. Put eggplant into bag and shake. Spray casserole dish with non-stick spray. Cover bottom of casserole dish with breaded eggplant. Pour tomato sauce over eggplant. Sprinkle cheese on top of eggplant. Bake, uncovered in 375 degree oven for 20 - 30 minutes or until cheese is bubbly. Remove from oven and sprinkle with Parmesan cheese.

Number of Servings: 4
Nutritional Analysis Per Serving:
Calories: 140
Fat: less than 1 gm (5%)
Fiber: 1 gm
Cholesterol: 1 mg
Saturated Fat: less than 1 gm
Beta Carotene: 1,260 I.U.
Vitamin C: 17 mg

Chili Mac

2 cups shredded Alpine Lace® FREE N' LEAN™ Cheddar Cheese

1 chopped Onion

1 chopped Green Pepper

3 shredded Carrots

2 pressed cloves of Garlic

1 15 oz. can of Kidney Beans

1 15 oz. can of Pinto Beans

2 15 oz. cans of Tomato Sauce

1 6 oz. can of Tomato Paste

1 tablespoon Chili Pepper

1 package Spaghetti

In large soup pot combine all ingredients except cheese, some onion and spaghetti. Be sure to wash beans in a colander first. Allow to simmer 2 to 3 hours. Remove chili from heat. Cook spaghetti until *al dente* then drain. Put spaghetti on individual plates. Spoon chili onto spaghetti Cover with cheese and remaining onion.

Number of Servings: 12
Nutritional Analysis Per Serving:
Calories: 233
Fat: less than 1 gm (3%)
Fiber: 10 gm
Cholesterol: -0-
Saturated Fat: less than 1 gm
Beta Carotene: 5,400 I.U.
Vitamin C: 30 mg

Cheese, Potato and Carrot Bake

1 cup shredded Alpine Lace® FREE N' LEAN™ Cheddar Cheese

4 peeled, thinly sliced Potatoes

4 peeled, shredded Carrots

1/2 cup thinly sliced Scallions

Salt and Pepper

Tear off several large sections of heavy-duty aluminum foil. Spray with non-stick spray. In center of each piece of foil layer potatoes, carrots, and scallions. Sprinkle with salt and pepper. Fold edges of foil over and seal completely, but leave enough space for steam to escape. Place in 350 degree oven for 45 - 50 minutes. Open each foil, add cheese, stir and re-seal for 2 minutes to allow cheese to melt.

Number of Servings: 4
Nutritional Analysis Per Serving:
Calories: 209
Fat: trace
Fiber: 2 gm
Cholesterol: -0-
Saturated Fat: -0-
Beta Carotene: 15,000 I.U.
Vitamin C: 30 mg

Twice-Baked Potatoes

4 baking Potatoes

1 cup shredded Alpine Lace® FREE N' LEAN™ American Cheese

1 thinly sliced Scallion

1/2 cup seasoned Bread Crumbs

Dash of Salt and Pepper

Scrub potatoes, stick with sharp knife, wrap individually in foil. Bake in 350 degree oven for 60 - 90 minutes. To check to see if potatoes are done, open one foil package and stick sharp knife into center, if it comes out easily potato is done. When all potatoes are done, remove from oven, unwrap foil and allow to cool for 5 to 10 minutes. Cut off the top of the potato lengthwise, scrape out top of potato, but try to leave potato skin in one piece. Scoop out the inside of the larger portion of each potato, leave skin intact, and place in large bowl, add cheese, scallion, salt and pepper. Stuff each potato skin with mixture. Sprinkle with bread crumbs. Add top portion of potato skin earlier set aside. Return to oven and bake for 10 minutes.

Number of Servings: 4
Nutritional Analysis Per Serving:
Calories: 214
Fat: trace
Fiber: 4 gm
Cholesterol: -0-
Saturated Fat: -0-
Beta Carotene: -0-
Vitamin C: 22 mg

Potato Skins

4 baking Potatoes

1 cup shredded Alpine Lace® FREE N' LEAN™ Cheddar Cheese

Dash of Salt and Pepper

Scrub potatoes, stick with sharp knife, wrap individually in foil. Bake in 350 degree oven for 60 - 90 minutes. To check to see if potatoes are done, open one foil package and stick sharp knife into center, if it comes out easily potato is done. When all potatoes are done, remove from oven, unwrap foil and allow to cool for 5 to 10 minutes. Cut the potatoes in half lengthwise, scrape small portion of center out of each potato half, but try to leave potato skin in one piece. Sprinkle inside of each potato half with salt and pepper. Place a generous amount of cheese on top of each hollowed out section. Return to oven and bake for 10 minutes or until cheese is melted.

Number of Servings: 4
Nutritional Analysis Per Serving:
Calories: 197
Fat: trace
Fiber: 4 gm
Cholesterol: -0-
Saturated Fat: -0-
Beta Carotene: -0-
Vitamin C: 20 mg

Scalloped Potatoes with Cheese

4 peeled, thinly sliced Potatoes
1 cup shredded Alpine Lace® FREE N' LEAN™ American Cheese
3 cups Skim Milk
1/2 cup chopped Scallion
2 tablespoons Butter Buds
2 tablespoons Flour
2 tablespoons seasoned Bread Crumbs
Salt and Pepper to taste

In a large skillet sprayed with non-stick spray, sauté scallions until tender. Add milk and allow to warm. Add flour, salt and pepper and stir well. After mixture is well combined, add cheese. Allow to simmer until mixture thickens and starts to bubble. While sauce is cooking, layer half of the potatoes in a casserole dish sprayed with non-stick spray. When sauce is finished cooking, pour half of the sauce over the potatoes in the dish, then layer the remaining potatoes over the sauce in the casserole dish. Pour any sauce in the pan over the potatoes. Sprinkle with bread crumbs. Cover and bake in 350 degree oven for 45 minutes. Uncover dish and continue to bake for 15 - 30 minutes or until top is golden brown.

Number of Servings: 6
Nutritional Analysis Per Serving:
Calories: 188
Fat: -0-
Fiber: 3 gm
Cholesterol: 2 mg
Saturated Fat: less than 1 gm
Beta Carotene: 750 I.U.
Vitamin C: 16 mg

Autumn Casserole with Cheese Sauce

1 medium size package of frozen Mixed Vegetables

1 cup shredded Alpine Lace® FREE N' LEAN™ American Cheese

2 cups quick-cooking Rice

1 sprig Thyme

1 teaspoon Oregano

1/2 thinly sliced Onion

Dash of Salt and Pepper

In a large bowl combine vegetables, cheese, rice, onion, salt and pepper. Mix well. Pour into casserole dish. Add 2 cups of warm water and stir until well distributed. Add thyme and oregano. Cover dish and place in 350 degree oven to bake for 45 minutes or until rice is fluffy.

Number of Servings: 8
Nutritional Analysis Per Serving:
Calories: 223
Fat: trace
Fiber: 2 gm
Cholesterol: -0-
Saturated Fat: -0-
Beta Carotene: 2,000 I.U.
Vitamin C: 3 mg

Broccoli, Carrot and Rice Casserole

2 cups Broccoli Flowerets
2 cups shredded Carrots
2 cups Instant Rice
2 cups shredded Alpine Lace® FREE N' LEAN™ Cheddar Cheese
1 cup Skim Milk
2 Egg Whites
1 thinly sliced Onion
1 cup seasoned Bread Crumbs
Salt and Pepper to taste

In a soup pot combine broccoli, carrots, rice and 5 cups of water. Bring to a boil. Reduce heat and simmer until rice is done. Remove from heat, add cheese, milk, eggs, onion, salt and pepper. Stir until well mixed. Pour into large casserole dish. Bake, uncovered in 350 degrees for 20 to 30 minutes. Remove from oven, sprinkle with bread crumbs. Return to oven for 2 minutes, then serve.

Number of Servings: 6
Nutritional Analysis Per Serving:
Calories: 265
Fat: trace
Fiber: 2 gm
Cholesterol: -0-
Saturated Fat: less than 1 gm
Beta Carotene: 11,600 I.U.
Vitamin C: 40 mg

Cheese and Vegetable Casserole

1 small package of frozen Cauliflower

1 small package of frozen Broccoli

1 small package of frozen Corn

1 cup shredded Alpine Lace® FREE N' LEAN™ Cheddar Cheese

1 10 3/4 oz. can of Mushroom Soup

1 cup seasoned Bread Crumbs

Cook and drain all vegetables, according to their packages, except corn. Pour vegetables into large bowl, add corn, mushroom soup and cheese. Mix well. Pour into large casserole dish sprayed with non-stick spray. Bake in 350 degree oven for 30 - 40 minutes. Remove from oven, sprinkle with bread crumbs, return to oven for 2 minutes, then serve.

Number of Servings: 8
Nutritional Analysis Per Serving:
Calories: 166
Fat: 2 gm (10%)
Fiber: 3 gm
Cholesterol: -0-
Saturated Fat: less than 1 gm
Beta Carotene: 1,000 I.U.
Vitamin C: 50 mg

Broccoli with Cheese Sauce

1 head of Broccoli

2 cups shredded Alpine Lace® FREE N' LEAN™ American Cheese

1 cup Skim Milk

1 tablespoon Flour

Cut broccoli flowerets and steam for 10 minutes. While broccoli is cooking, warm milk slowly in saucepan over low heat. Toss cheese with flour in bowl then add to milk in saucepan. Allow cheese and milk to simmer until mixture is completely smooth. When broccoli and cheese are finished cooking, place broccoli on serving dishes, spoon cheese sauce over broccoli.

Number of Servings: 4
Nutritional Analysis Per Serving:
Calories: 208
Fat: -0-
Fiber: 4 gm
Cholesterol: -0-
Saturated Fat: -0-
Beta Carotene: 5,300 I.U.
Vitamin C: 50 mg

Baked Tomatoes

4 plump Tomatoes

4 slices Alpine Lace® FREE N' LEAN™ Mozzarella Cheese

2 tablespoons Italian Seasonings

Slice tomatoes in half. Sprinkle with seasonings. Place one slice of cheese on each half of tomato. Place in 200 degree oven and allow to bake for 5 - 10 minutes or until cheese is lightly browned.

Number of Servings: 4
Nutritional Analysis Per Serving:
Calories: 60
Fat: -0-
Fiber: 2 gm
Cholesterol: -0-
Saturated Fat: -0-
Beta Carotene: 1,375 I.U.
Vitamin C: 22 mg

Cheese Stuffed Peppers

6 Green Peppers

1 cup Alpine Lace® FREE N' LEAN™ American Cheese

1 finely chopped Onion

2 diced Tomatoes

1 cup cooked Brown Rice

1 teaspoon Worcestershire Sauce

Cut the top off of each green pepper. Scrape out seeds and membranes from inside each pepper and discard. Chop up the usable part of each top and set aside 1/4 cup. Using a large soup pot, boil whole peppers in water for 5 minutes. Remove and drain upside down. While peppers are cooling, combine cheese, onion, tomatoes, rice, chopped green pepper and worcestershire sauce in large bowl and mix well. Stuff mixture into each hollowed out pepper. Place peppers right side up in casserole dish, cover and bake in 350 degree oven for 30 - 40 minutes.

Number of Servings: 6
Nutritional Analysis Per Serving:
Calories: 110
Fat: trace
Fiber: 2 gm
Cholesterol: -0-
Saturated Fat: -0-
Beta Carotene: 853 I.U.
Vitamin C: 105 mg

Cheddar Cheese Bread

2 cups all-purpose Flour
2 cups whole wheat Flour
2 cups shredded Alpine Lace® FREE N' LEAN™ Cheddar Cheese
1/4 cup Sugar
1 teaspoon Salt
1 package of Active Dry Yeast
1 Egg White

In a large bowl combine 1 1/2 cups of flour and yeast. In a small sauce pan mix 2 1/2 cups of water, cheese, sugar and salt. Cook until it starts to gently simmer. Remove from heat and allow to cool for 10 minutes. Add cheese mixture to flour and yeast, mix on low speed with electric mixer. Add egg and continue to mix on higher speed. Using a spoon, mix as much additional flour as possible into dough. Pour dough out of bowl onto well floured surface. Kneed dough until stiff yet elastic, 5 to 8 minutes. Shape into two balls, place each in a bowl sprayed with non-stick spray turn once, cover, place in warm place and let rise until double in size (not longer than an hour). Turn each ball into a loaf pan and bake in 350 degree oven for 30 or 40 minutes or until golden brown. If top of loaf starts to get too brown, cover with tin foil and allow to continue baking until done. Cool on wire rack. Makes 2 loaves.

Number of Servings: 12
Nutritional Analysis Per Serving:
Calories: 190
Fat: less than 1 gm (2%)
Fiber: less than 1 gm
Cholesterol: -0-
Saturated Fat: -0-
Beta Carotene: -0-
Vitamin C: -0-

Cheddar Cheese Corn Bread

1 cup Corn Meal

1 cup all-purpose Flour

1 cup shredded Alpine Lace® FREE N' LEAN™ Cheddar Cheese

1/3 cup Sugar

3 teaspoons Baking Powder

1 cup Skim Milk

2 Egg Whites

Dash of Salt

In a large bowl mix together corn meal, flour, sugar, baking powder and salt. Add egg whites and milk and stir until smooth (do not stir too much). Add cheese and mix briefly. Pour into 9x9x2 inch baking pan sprayed with non-stick spray. Bake in 425 degree oven for 20 minutes or until golden brown.

Number of Servings: 8
Nutritional Analysis Per Serving:
Calories: 176
Fat: less than 1 gm (2%)
Fiber: 2 gm
Cholesterol: -0-
Saturated Fat: -0-
Beta Carotene: 138 I.U.
Vitamin C: trace

Cheddar Cheese Muffins

2 cups all-purpose Flour

3/4 cup shredded Alpine Lace® FREE N' LEAN™ Cheddar Cheese

1/3 cup Sugar

3 teaspoons Baking Powder

1 cup Skim Milk

1 Egg White

Dash of Salt

In a large bowl mix together flour, sugar, baking powder and salt. Add milk and egg white. Stir until smooth, but not too much. Add cheese and mix well. Put baking cups into muffin tin and spoon batter into baking cups. Bake in 375 degree oven for 20 minutes or until golden brown.

Number of Servings: 12
Nutritional Analysis Per Serving:
Calories: 108
Fat: less than 1 gm (1%)
Fiber: 1 gm
Cholesterol: trace
Saturated Fat: -0-
Beta Carotene: 41 I.U.
Vitamin C: trace

Apple Cheese Cobbler

6 peeled, thinly sliced cooking Apples

1 cup shredded Alpine Lace® FREE N' LEAN™ Cheddar Cheese

1 cup Sugar

1/4 cup Flour

1 teaspoon Ground Cinnamon

1 teaspoon Ground Allspice

1/4 cup Water

In a large bowl combine sugar, flour, cinnamon and allspice. Set aside 1/3 cup of mixture. Add apples and cheese to the bulk of the sugar mixture and toss well. Add water and stir well. Spoon into individual cobbler baking dishes or deep baking dish. Sprinkle with sugar mixture previously set aside. Bake in 350 degree oven for 30 minutes.

Number of Servings: 8
Nutritional Analysis Per Serving:
Calories: 178
Fat: -0-
Fiber: 1 gm
Cholesterol: -0-
Saturated Fat: -0-
Beta Carotene: 375 I.U.
Vitamin C: 6 mg

Side Dishes

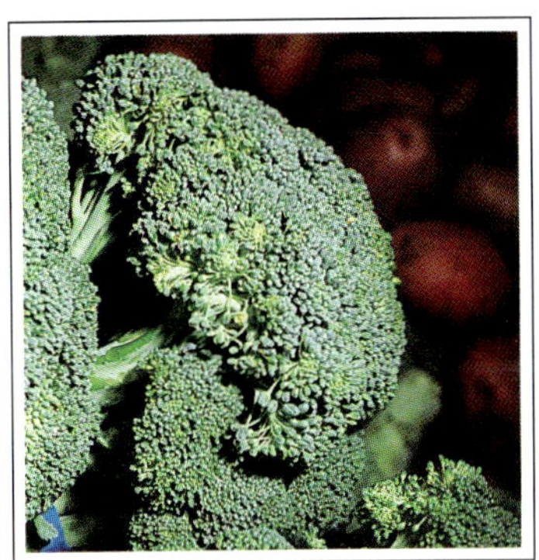

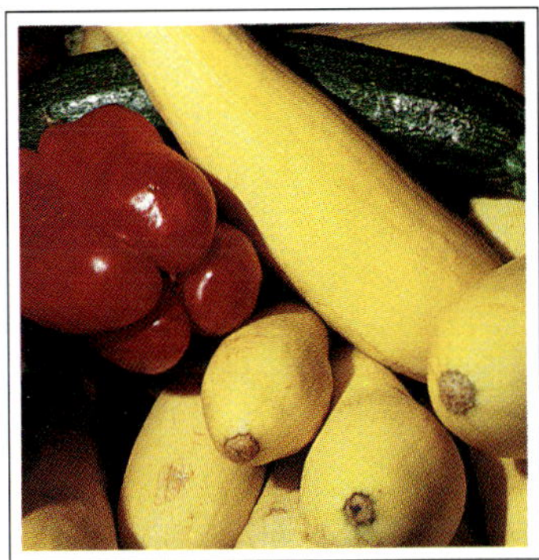

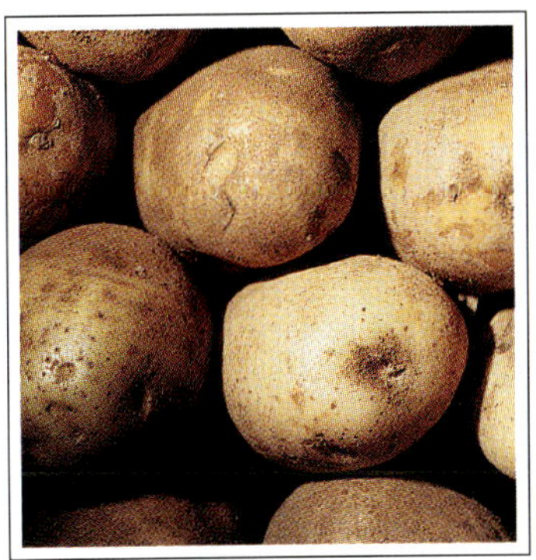

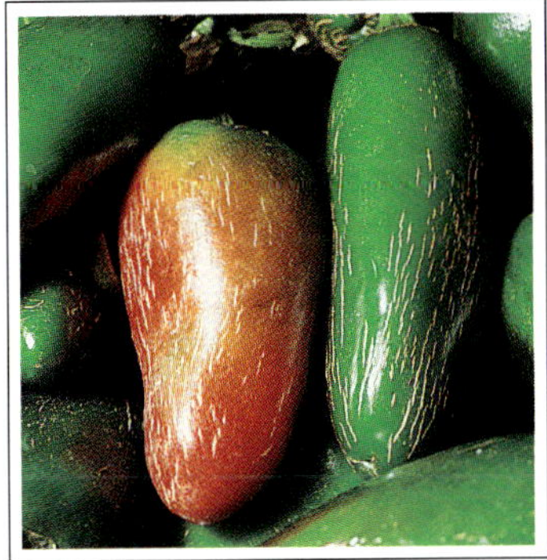

Bread Stuffing

10 pieces toasted, cubed Whole Wheat Bread

1 shredded Carrot

1 finely chopped stalk of Celery

1 finely chopped Onion

2 cubes Chicken Bouillon
(dissolved in one cup warm water)

1 tablespoon Olive Oil

In a skillet, warm olive oil on low-medium heat. Add onion, sauté until soft. Put bread in a large bowl, add carrot and celery, toss well. Dissolve bouillon in one cup of warm water. Add broth made with bouillon and onions to bowl and stir well. Put in baking dish, cover and bake in 350 degree oven for 20 minutes. Remove from oven, stir and put in serving bowl.

Number of Servings: 6
Nutritional Analysis Per Serving:
Calories: 154
Fat: 4 gm (24%)
Fiber: 1 gm
Cholesterol: -0-
Saturated Fat: 1 gm
Beta Carotene: 3,300 I.U.
Vitamin C: 4 mg

Bread Stuffing with Raisins

10 pieces toasted, cubed Whole Wheat Bread

1 tablespoon Olive Oil

3 shredded Carrots

1 finely chopped Onion

1 cup Raisins

2 cubes Chicken Bouillon

2 teaspoons Cinnamon

In a skillet, warm olive oil over medium heat. Add onion, sauté until soft. Put bread in a large bowl, add carrots and raisins, toss well. Dissolve bouillon in 1 cup of warm water. Add broth and onions to bowl, stir well. Add cinnamon, one teaspoon at a time and stir well. Put in baking dish, cover and bake in 350 degree oven for 20 minutes. Remove from oven, stir and put in serving bowl.

Number of Servings: 8
Nutritional Analysis Per Serving:
Calories: 175
Fat: 3 gm (16%)
Fiber: 2 gm
Cholesterol: trace
Saturated Fat: less than 1 gm
Beta Carotene: 7,600 I.U.
Vitamin C: 5 mg

Baked Beans

1 16 oz. can of Beans in Tomato Sauce

1 15 oz. can of Navy Beans (rinsed and drained)

1 15 oz. can of Garbanzo Beans (rinsed and drained)

1 chopped Onion

1/4 cup Brown Sugar (dissolved in 1 cup warm water)

2 tablespoons Mustard

1 tablespoon Worcestershire Sauce

In a large bowl combine all above ingredients one at a time mixing well before adding the next. When all are mixed well, put in a large casserole dish and bake in 350 degree oven for 1 hour.

Number of Servings: 8
Nutritional Analysis Per Serving:
Calories: 193
Fat: 1 gm (6%)
Fiber: 7 gm
Cholesterol: -0-
Saturated Fat: less than 1 gm
Beta Carotene: -0-
Vitamin C: 6 mg

Baked Beets

1 16 oz. can of sliced Beets

2 tablespoons Brown Sugar

1 tablespoon Cinnamon

Arrange beets in layers on the bottom of a shallow casserole dish. Add cinnamon and brown sugar to 1/2 cup warm water, stir then pour over beets. Cover and bake in preheated 350 degree oven for 30 - 40 minutes, or until beets are soft.

Number of Servings: 4
Nutritional Analysis Per Serving:
Calories: 50
Fat: trace
Fiber: 1 gm
Cholesterol: -0-
Saturated Fat: -0-
Beta Carotene: 9 I.U.
Vitamin C: 5 mg

Baked Broccoli

1 head of Broccoli

3 shredded Carrots

1 10 3/4 oz. can of condensed Cream of Mushroom Soup

1 cup Bread Crumbs

Cut broccoli into stalks with flowerets. Rinse and drain well. Toss broccoli and carrots in large bowl, put into casserole dish. Mix mushroom soup with 2 cups of warm water. Cover broccoli and carrots with mushroom soup. Sprinkle bread crumbs over broccoli. Cover and bake in 350 degree oven for 30 - 40 minutes.

Number of Servings: 4
Nutritional Analysis Per Serving:
Calories: 140
Fat: 5 gm (32%)
Fiber: 2 gm
Cholesterol: 1 mg
Saturated Fat: 1 gm
Beta Carotene: 16,000 I.U.
Vitamin C: 53 mg

Couscous

2 cups of Couscous grain

2 teaspoons Olive Oil

1 chopped Onion

1 pressed clove of Garlic

2 chopped Tomatoes

1 diced Green Pepper

3 shredded Carrots

In a large skillet, warm olive oil over medium heat. Add onion and garlic, sauté until soft. Add tomatoes, green pepper and carrots. Cook until vegetables are tender, about 10 minutes. Add vegetables to prepared couscous and mix well.

Number of Servings: 6
Nutritional Analysis Per Serving:
Calories: 202
Fat: less than 1 gm (3%)
Fiber: 2 gm
Cholesterol: -0-
Saturated Fat: less than 1 gm
Beta Carotene: 10,600 I.U.
Vitamin C: 29 mg

Moroccan Carrots

1 pound of thinly sliced Carrots
4 tablespoons Olive Oil
1/4 cup Balsamic Vinegar
3/4 cup Red Wine Vinegar
4 tablespoons Paprika
4 tablespoons Ground Cumin
2 pressed cloves of Garlic
2 teaspoons Ground Cloves
4 tablespoons Minced Parsley

Boil carrots in water until crisp yet tender. While carrots are cooking, combine olive oil, balsamic vinegar, red wine vinegar, paprika and cumin in container. Shake well. When carrots have finished cooking, drain and place in air tight container, pour dressing over carrots, then sprinkle with garlic, cloves, parsley. Cover and marinate 2 - 3 days. (Note: Very few grams of fat will ultimately be absorbed by the finished carrots.)

Number of Servings: 10
Nutritional Analysis Per Serving:
Calories: 42
Fat: 1 gm (30%)
Fiber: 1 gm
Cholesterol: -0-
Saturated Fat: less than 1 gm
Beta Carotene: 20,000 I.U.
Vitamin C: 5 mg

Lemon Carrots

10 thinly sliced Carrots

1 Lemon

1 tablespoon Lemon Juice

Place carrots in bowl. In a separate bowl, grate lemon rind then set aside. Cut lemon into pieces and squeeze juice out over carrots. Add additional lemon juice to carrots and stir. Add lemon rind and stir well. Cover and allow to marinate overnight.

Number of Servings: 10
Nutritional Analysis Per Serving:
Calories: 32
Fat: -0-
Fiber: 1 gm
Cholesterol: -0-
Saturated Fat: -0-
Beta Carotene: 20,000 I.U.
Vitamin C: 10 mg

Italian Cauliflower

1 head Cauliflower

1 tablespoon Olive Oil

2 tablespoons White Vinegar

2 tablespoons Italian Seasoning

1 sliced Green Pepper

1 sliced Red Pepper

Cut cauliflower into flowerets then steam until tender. While cauliflower is steaming, mix together olive oil, vinegar and seasoning. When cauliflower is finished cooking, rinse with cool water and drain. Put into bowl, pour on seasoning mixture and stir well. Add peppers and stir again. Store in covered container and marinate overnight or longer.

Number of Servings: 4
Nutritional Analysis Per Serving:
Calories: 55
Fat: 4 gm (57%)
Fiber: 1 gm
Cholesterol: -0-
Saturated Fat: less than 1 gm
Beta Carotene: 1,200 I.U.
Vitamin C: 100 mg

Creamy Cucumbers

4 peeled, diced Cucumbers

1 finely chopped sweet Onion

1 pint Non-Fat Yogurt

3 tablespoons chopped Dill

Place cucumbers in bowl. Stir in yogurt. Add onion, stir well. Place in serving bowl and sprinkle with dill.

Number of Servings: 4
Nutritional Analysis Per Serving:
Calories: 70
Fat: trace
Fiber: 2 gm
Cholesterol: 1 mg
Saturated Fat: less than 1 gm
Beta Carotene: 55 I.U.
Vitamin C: 9 mg

Baked French Fries

3 peeled Potatoes

2 teaspoons Olive Oil

Salt to taste

Cut potatoes into thin strips lengthwise. Put in bowl, sprinkle with olive oil and toss. Place on cookie sheet sprayed with non-stick spray. Cook in 350 degree oven for 10 minutes, remove from oven, turn potatoes over and return to oven until golden brown. Remove from oven and sprinkle lightly with salt.

Number of Servings: 4
Nutritional Analysis Per Serving:
Calories: 175
Fat: 1 gm (6%)
Fiber: 2 gm
Cholesterol: -0-
Saturated Fat: trace
Beta Carotene: -0-
Vitamin C: 15 mg

Spiced Green Beans

1 pound cut, cleaned Green Beans

1 15 oz. can of Tomato Sauce

1 teaspoon Tabasco Sauce

1 teaspoon Basil

Cook green beans until tender yet crisp in large pot of boiling water. While green beans are cooking, combine tomato sauce, Tabasco Sauce and basil in sauce pan and warm over medium heat. Cover and simmer sauce until beans are done. When beans have finished cooking, drain, then return to pot. Pour sauce over beans. Simmer together for 10 minutes then serve.

Number of Servings: 4
Nutritional Analysis Per Serving:
Calories: 60
Fat: -0-
Fiber: 2 gm
Cholesterol: -0-
Saturated Fat: trace
Beta Carotene: 1,600 I.U.
Vitamin C: 50 mg

Lima Beans in Garlic Seasoning

1 package of Lima Beans

4 pressed cloves of Garlic

1 tablespoon Olive Oil

Garlic Salt

In a large skillet warm olive oil over low heat. Sauté garlic in oil briefly then add Lima beans. Cover and allow to sauté for 15 - 20 minutes, stirring frequently. Remove from heat, sprinkle lightly with garlic salt then serve.

Number of Servings: 4
Nutritional Analysis Per Serving:
Calories: 220
Fat: 4 gm (18%)
Fiber: 4 gm
Cholesterol: -0-
Saturated Fat: less than 1 gm
Beta Carotene: 300 I.U.
Vitamin C: 22 mg

Curried Onions

3 sliced Onions

1 tablespoon Olive Oil

2 tablespoons Curry Powder

In a large skillet warm olive oil on low heat. Add curry powder and stir well. Add onions. Cook for 10 minutes, or until onions are limp, stirring constantly. Serve over a bed of rice or baked potato.

Number of Servings: 4
Nutritional Analysis Per Serving:
Calories: 70
Fat: 3 gm (45%)
Fiber: 1 gm
Cholesterol: -0-
Saturated Fat: less than 1 gm
Beta Carotene: 30 I.U.
Vitamin C: 10 mg

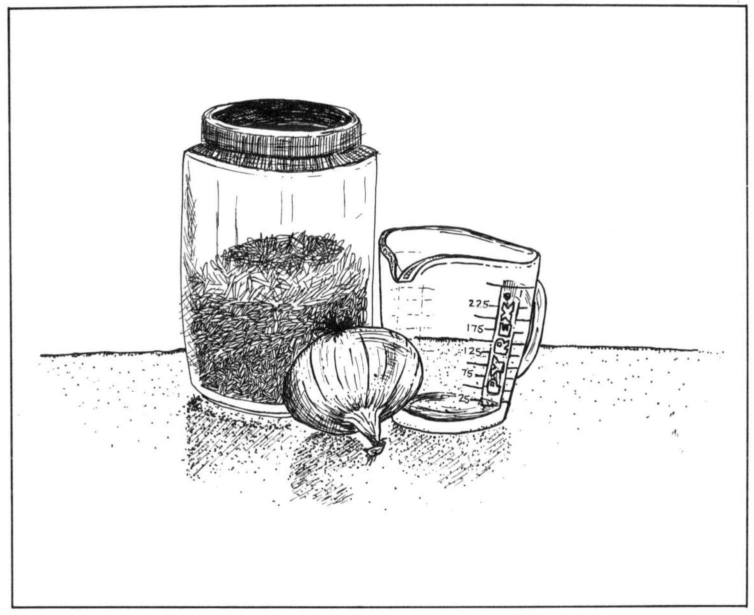

Pilaf

Pilaf

1 cup long grain Rice

1 tablespoon Olive Oil

1 cup short Pasta or Orzo

1 chopped Onion

3 cubes Chicken Bouillon

Sauté onion in olive oil in skillet on low heat. When onions are soft add rice and stir often. While rice is cooking, dissolve bouillon in 2 cups of water. Add broth and pasta to rice, cover skillet and allow to simmer for 20 minutes or until all of the broth is absorbed and rice and pasta are tender. Add more water if necessary. Salt and pepper to taste.

Number of Servings: 4
Nutritional Analysis Per Serving:
Calories: 185
Fat: 4 gm (19%)
Fiber: less than 1 gm
Cholesterol: less than 1 mg
Saturated Fat: less than 1 gm
Beta Carotene: -0-
Vitamin C: 4 mg

Stuffed Peppers

6 Green Peppers

1 chopped sweet Onion

1 16 oz. can of Plum Tomatoes

1/2 cup long grain Rice

1 tablespoon Olive Oil

1 teaspoon Basil

1 teaspoon Oregano

Cut tops off of green peppers. Place peppers in large pot of boiling water for 5 minutes. Remove and drain upside down. Cut the useable portion of the pepper tops into small pieces and set aside. In a skillet, sauté the onion and pepper picces in olive oil until tender. Add undrained tomatoes, uncooked rice, basil and oregano to skillet. Bring to a boil then reduce heat. Cover and simmer 15 - 20 minutes or until rice is tender. Remove from heat and stuff mixture into green peppers. Place peppers in covered baking dish. Bake in 350 degree oven for 30 minutes.

Number of Servings: 6
Nutritional Analysis Per Serving:
Calories: 140
Fat: 4 gm (24%)
Fiber: 2 gm
Cholesterol: -0-
Saturated Fat: less than 1 gm
Beta Carotene: 2,000 I.U.
Vitamin C: 165 mg

Bavarian Potatoes

20 cleaned, halved New Potatoes

2 cups Low-Fat Cottage Cheese

1 cup Non-Fat Plain Yogurt

1 bunch of finely chopped Scallions

Salt and Pepper to taste

Paprika

Steam potatoes for 20 minutes, or until done (test with fork). While potatoes are cooking, mix together cottage cheese, yogurt and scallions. Remove potatoes from heat and drain. Put in serving bowl and add cottage cheese mixture. Mix well. Sprinkle with salt, pepper and paprika.

Number of Servings: 10
Nutritional Analysis Per Serving:
Calories: 200
Fat: 1 gm (4%)
Fiber: 2 gm
Cholesterol: 10 mg
Saturated Fat: 1 gm
Beta Carotene: 85 I.U.
Vitamin C: 33 mg

Garlic Potatoes

6 peeled, cubed boiling Potatoes

6 pressed cloves of Garlic

1 tablespoon Olive Oil

Garlic salt

Boil potatoes until done (test with fork). While potatoes are cooking, sauté garlic in olive oil on low heat briefly. When potatoes and garlic are finished put both into a bowl and mash. Add garlic salt to taste.

Number of Servings: 6
Nutritional Analysis Per Serving:
Calories: 240
Fat: 2 gm (9%)
Fiber: 2 gm
Cholesterol: -0-
Saturated Fat: less than 1 gm
Beta Carotene: -0-
Vitamin C: 20 mg

"Fried" Potatoes

2 thinly sliced Potatoes

1 finely chopped Onion

2 teaspoons Olive Oil

Salt and Pepper to taste

Heat olive oil slowly in skillet. Add onion and potatoes. Stir frequently, on low heat, allowing to brown. Cook for approximately 15 - 20 minutes or until done. Salt and pepper to taste.

Number of Servings: 2
Nutritional Analysis Per Serving:
Calories: 287
Fat: 4 gm (14%)
Fiber: 2 gm
Cholesterol: -0-
Saturated Fat: less than 1 gm
Beta Carotene: -0-
Vitamin C: 26 mg

Marvelous Mashed Potatoes

6 peeled and cubed boiling Potatoes

1/2 cup Skim Milk

1/2 cup Low-Fat Cottage Cheese

Salt and Pepper to taste

Boil potatoes until done (test with fork). While potatoes are cooking, mix together milk and cottage cheese. When potatoes are finished cooking remove from heat, drain and place in bowl. Mash potatoes until fairly smooth. Add cottage cheese mixture and continue to mash until smooth. Add salt and pepper to taste.

Number of Servings: 8
Nutritional Analysis Per Serving:
Calories: 180
Fat: less than 1 gm (10%)
Fiber: 1 gm
Cholesterol: 1 mg
Saturated Fat: less than 1 gm
Beta Carotene: 41 I.U.
Vitamin C: 15 mg

Hearty Stuffed Potatoes

4 cleaned, baking Potatoes

1 finely chopped Onion

3 pressed cloves of Garlic

1 tablespoon Olive Oil

2 tablespoons Feta Cheese

2 tablespoons minced Chives

Bake potatoes for 60 - 90 minutes in oven. While potatoes are cooking sauté onion and garlic in olive oil until soft. When potatoes are done cut each potato in half lengthwise. Scoop out center of each potato, keep potato skin intact, and set in bowl. Add onion, garlic, feta cheese and chives, mix well. Stuff potato skins with mixture, being careful not to tear potato skin. Bake in 350 degree oven for 15 minutes. Sprinkle with additional chives when finished baking.

Number of Servings: 4
Nutritional Analysis Per Serving:
Calories: 280
Fat: 5 gm (16%)
Fiber: 2 gm
Cholesterol: 6 mg
Saturated Fat: 1 gm
Beta Carotene: 32 I.U.
Vitamin C: 23 mg

Italian Stuffed Potatoes

4 cleaned, baking Potatoes

1 finely chopped Onion

3 pressed cloves of Garlic

1 teaspoon Olive Oil

2 tablespoons Basil

2 tablespoons Oregano

1 tablespoon sweet Vinegar

1 tablespoon Italian Seasonings

Bake potatoes for 60 - 90 minutes in oven. While potatoes are cooking sauté onion and garlic in olive oil until soft. When potatoes are done cut each potato in half lengthwise. Scoop out center of each potato, keep potato skin intact, and set in bowl. Add onion and garlic to potatoes in bowl, mix well. Add basil, oregano, seasonings and vinegar, mix well. Stuff potato skins with mixture, being careful not to tear potato skin. Bake in 350 degree oven for 15 minutes.

Number of Servings: 4
Nutritional Analysis Per Serving:
Calories: 245
Fat: 1 gm (5%)
Fiber: 2 gm
Cholesterol: -0-
Saturated Fat: less than 1 gm
Beta Carotene: trace
Vitamin C: 25 mg

Vegetable Garden Stuffed Potatoes

4 cleaned, baking Potatoes

1 finely chopped Onion

3 pressed cloves of Garlic

1 tablespoon Olive Oil

1 shredded Carrot

1 cup Broccoli flowerets

1/2 cup finely chopped Red Pepper

Bake potatoes for 60 - 90 minutes in oven. While potatoes are cooking sauté onion and garlic in olive oil until soft. When potatoes are done cut each potato in half lengthwise. Scoop out center of each potato, keep potato skin intact, and set in bowl. Add onion and garlic to potatoes in bowl, mix well. Add carrot, broccoli and red pepper, stirring well after adding each. Stuff potato skins with mixture, being careful not to tear potato skin. Sprinkle with salt and pepper. Serve while mixture is warm.

Number of Servings: 4
Nutritional Analysis Per Serving:
Calories: 296
Fat: 3.5 gm (11%)
Fiber: 3 gm
Cholesterol: -0-
Saturated Fat: less than 1 gm
Beta Carotene: 6,600 I.U.
Vitamin C: 67 mg

Mexican Rice

2 cups medium grain cooked Rice

1 8 oz. can of Tomato Sauce

1 finely chopped Green Pepper

1 finely chopped Red Pepper

Warm tomato sauce in sauce pan. Add rice and pepper. Continue to cook just until peppers are slightly tender.

Number of Servings: 4
Nutritional Analysis Per Serving:
Calories: 140
Fat: trace
Fiber: 1 gm
Cholesterol: -0-
Saturated Fat: less than 1 gm
Beta Carotene: 2,000 I.U.
Vitamin C: 65 mg

Country Spinach

1 pound uncooked Spinach

1 bunch chopped Scallions

3 shredded Carrots

1 pressed clove of Garlic

1 tablespoon Olive Oil

Cook spinach in a large pot of boiling water, do not overcook. Drain when finished. While spinach is cooking, sauté garlic in olive oil briefly on low heat. Leave in skillet but remove from heat when finished cooking. Add drained spinach to skillet and stir so that the spinach absorbs all of the garlic and olive oil flavor. Place spinach in mixing bowl and add scallions and carrots, mix together well.

Number of Servings: 4
Nutritional Analysis Per Serving:
Calories: 60
Fat: 3.5 gm (52%)
Fiber: 2 gm
Cholesterol: -0-
Saturated Fat: less than 1 gm
Beta Carotene: 17,000 I.U.
Vitamin C: 25 mg

Squash

1 Acorn Squash

2 tablespoons Honey

1/2 teaspoon Nutmeg

1/2 teaspoon Cinnamon

Cut squash in half and bake for 45 minutes or microwave for 10 - 15 minutes. While squash is cooking mix together honey, nutmeg and cinnamon. Just before serving heat the honey mixture and pour over squash. Serve warm.

Number of Servings: 4
Nutritional Analysis Per Serving:
Calories: 72
Fat: trace
Fiber: 8 gm
Cholesterol: -0-
Saturated Fat: trace
Beta Carotene: 3,645 I.U.
Vitamin C: 5 mg

Baked Sweet Potatoes

3 peeled, cubed Sweet Potatoes

2 tablespoons Honey

2 tablespoons Brown Sugar

1 teaspoon Cinnamon

1 teaspoon Nutmeg

Mini-Marshmallows

Boil sweet potatoes until done (test with fork). Remove potatoes from heat, drain well and mash. Add honey, brown sugar, cinnamon and nutmeg then mix well. Turn mixture into casserole dish sprayed with non-stick spray. Sprinkle with several marshmallows. Bake in 350 degree oven until marshmallows melt and turn lightly browned.

Number of Servings: 4
Nutritional Analysis Per Serving:
Calories: 180
Fat: less than 1 gm (4%)
Fiber: 2 gm
Cholesterol: -0-
Saturated Fat: -0-
Beta Carotene: 7,000 I.U.
Vitamin C: 5 mg

Stuffed Tomatoes

4 Tomatoes

1 cup cooked Spinach

2 finely chopped Scallions

1 cup Low-Fat Cottage Cheese

Salt and Pepper to taste

Scoop out center of tomato, being careful to leave skin intact. Set tomato parts aside separately. In a mixing bowl combine spinach, scallions, cottage cheese, salt and pepper. Stuff tomato skins with mixture and serve while stuffing is warm.

Number of Servings: 4
Nutritional Analysis Per Serving:
Calories: 90
Fat: 1 gm (10%)
Fiber: 1 gm
Cholesterol: 5 mg
Saturated Fat: less than 1 gm
Beta Carotene: 5,100 I.U.
Vitamin C: 33 mg

Vegetable Medley

2 cubed, boiling Potatoes

4 shredded Carrots

2 thinly sliced Zucchini

1 pound Spinach

2 15 oz. cans of Tomato Sauce

1 teaspoon Curry Powder

1 teaspoon Worcestershire Sauce

Put all of the above ingredients in soup pot, except spinach, with 4 cups of water. Allow to cook slowly on low heat for 45 minutes, stirring often. Add spinach 5 minutes before serving.

Number of Servings: 4
Nutritional Analysis Per Serving:
Calories: 181
Fat: less than 1 gm (3%)
Fiber: 2 gm
Cholesterol: -0-
Saturated Fat: less than 1 gm
Beta Carotene: 25,000 I.U.
Vitamin C: 70 mg

Pan "Fried" Zucchini

2 thinly sliced Zucchini

1 Egg White

1 cup Skim Milk

1 cup Corn Meal

4 tablespoons Safflower Oil

Combine egg white and skim milk. Soak sliced zucchini in mixture. Put corn meal in paper bag. Put zucchini, without liquid, in paper bag and shake well. Heat oil in skillet and add zucchini, small amounts at a time. Cook for 5 minutes on each side. Drain on paper towels.

Number of Servings: 4
Nutritional Analysis Per Serving:
Calories: 271
Fat: 15 gm (51%)
Fiber: 1 gm
Cholesterol: 1 mg
Saturated Fat: 1 gm
Beta Carotene: 5,000 I.U.
Vitamin C: 3 mg

Spicy Zucchini

3 thinly sliced Zucchini

2 grated Carrots

3 sliced Tomatoes

1 15 oz. can of Tomato Sauce

1 finely chopped Onion

2 stalks of Celery, chopped

1 finely chopped Green Pepper

1 finely chopped Red Pepper

2 tablespoons Basil

2 tablespoons Oregano

1 teaspoon Tabasco Sauce

Combine 2 tomatoes, tomato sauce, onion, celery, peppers, basil, oregano, and Tabasco Sauce in large mixing bowl. Using masher, combine ingredients. Layer zucchini, carrots, and remaining tomato in bottom of casserole dish. Pour sauce over layers. Cover and bake in 350 degree oven for 30 - 40 minutes. Uncover and bake an additional 15 minutes.

Number of Servings: 4
Nutritional Analysis Per Serving:
Calories: 140
Fat: -0-
Fiber: 3 gm
Cholesterol: -0-
Saturated Fat: -0-
Beta Carotene: 15,000 I.U.
Vitamin C: 100 mg

Desserts and Baked Goods

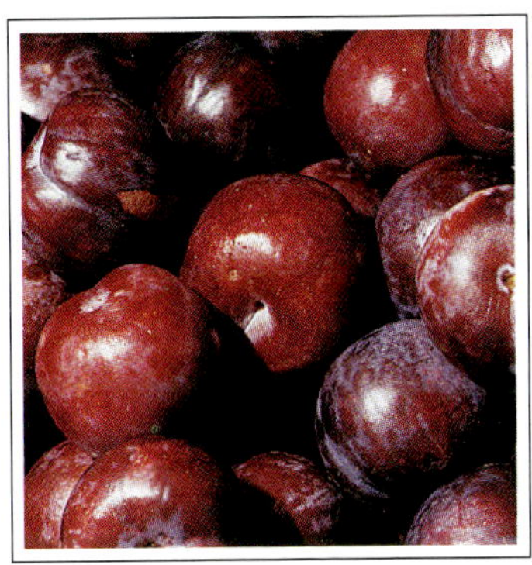
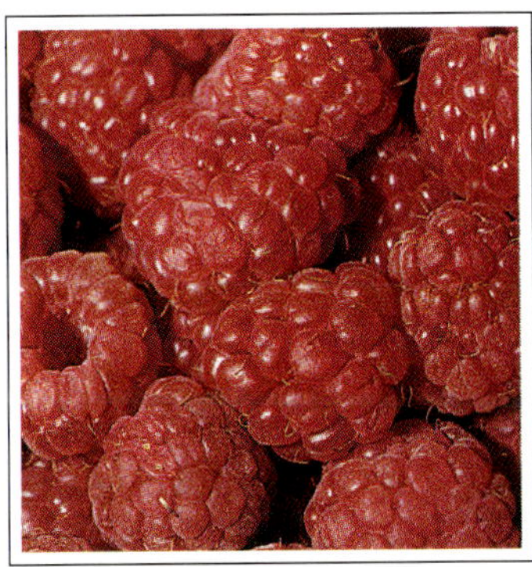
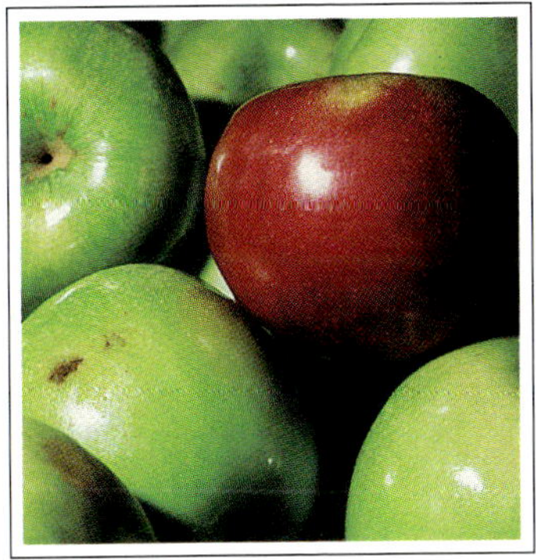
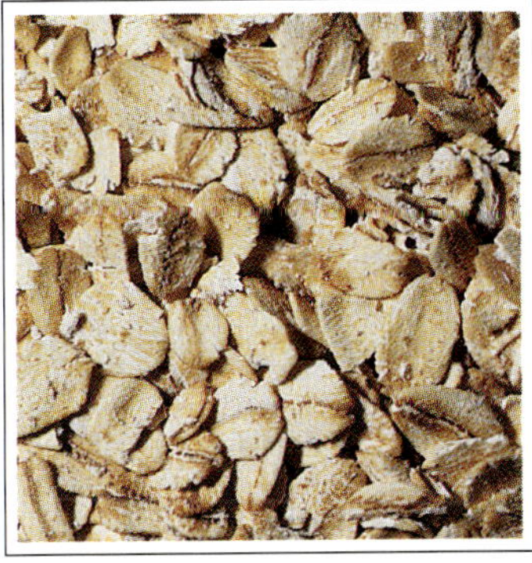

Apple Crisp

6 sliced Apples

2 cups Rolled Oats

5 tablespoons Flour

1/4 teaspoon Cinnamon

1/4 teaspoon Nutmeg

1/4 teaspoon Cloves

1 8 oz. can of crushed Pineapple

Place apples in shallow baking dish sprayed with non-stick spray. Sprinkle with cinnamon, nutmeg and cloves. Spoon pineapple over apple. Combine oats with flour and sprinkle over apples and pineapple. Cover and bake in 350 degree oven for 40 - 50 minutes.

Number of Servings: 8
Nutritional Analysis Per Serving:
Calories: 115
Fat: less than 1 gm (4%)
Fiber: 2 gm
Cholesterol: -0-
Saturated Fat: less than 1 gm
Beta Carotene: 150 I.U.
Vitamin C: 9 mg

Applesauce Spice Cake

1 16 oz. can of Applesauce

1 cup Sugar

2 Egg Whites

2 1/2 cups all-purpose Flour

1 1/2 teaspoons Baking Soda

1/4 teaspoon Baking Powder

1 teaspoon Ground Cinnamon

1 teaspoon Allspice

Combine flour, baking soda, baking powder, cinnamon and allspice. Sift together. Add sugar and stir well. Add egg whites and mix together until well combined. Add applesauce and beat until creamy. Pour into large cake pan sprayed with non-stick spray. Bake in 350 degree oven for 40 - 45 minutes or until done.

Number of Servings: 10
Nutritional Analysis Per Serving:
Calories: 200
Fat: less than 1 gm (2%)
Fiber: trace
Cholesterol: -0-
Saturated Fat: -0-
Beta Carotene: 14 I.U.
Vitamin C: 1 mg

Stuffed Baked Apples

6 cored Apples

2 cups Rolled Oats

5 tablespoons Flour

1/4 teaspoon Cinnamon

1/4 teaspoon Nutmeg

1/4 teaspoon Cloves

1 cup Raisins

Combine oats, flour, cinnamon, nutmeg, cloves and raisins in bowl. Add 1/2 cup of water and mix well. Fill cored apples with mixture. Cover and bake in shallow dish with 1/4-inch of water in 350 degree oven for 45 minutes.

Number of Servings: 8
Nutritional Analysis Per Serving:
Calories: 150
Fat: less than 1 gm (4%)
Fiber: 2 gm
Cholesterol: -0-
Saturated Fat: less than 1 gm
Beta Carotene: 63 I.U.
Vitamin C: 6 mg

Apple and Yam Bake

6 peeled and cubed Apples

2 peeled and sliced Yams

1/4 teaspoon Cinnamon

1/4 teaspoon Nutmeg

1/4 teaspoon Cloves

1/2 cup Sugar

Combine cinnamon, nutmeg, cloves and sugar. Mix well then divide in half. Place apples and yams in bowl. Pour half of the spices over apples and yams and mix well. Spray casserole dish with non-stick spray and pour in apples and yams. Sprinkle remaining mixed spices on top. Cover and bake in 350 degree oven for 45 minutes.

Number of Servings: 8
Nutritional Analysis Per Serving:
Calories: 125
Fat: less than 1 gm (2%)
Fiber: 2 gm
Cholesterol: -0-
Saturated Fat: less than 1 gm
Beta Carotene: 2,000 I.U.
Vitamin C: 11 mg

Apple Turnovers

4 thinly sliced Apples
1/4 cup Sugar
1/4 teaspoon Cinnamon
1/4 teaspoon Nutmeg
1/4 teaspoon Cloves
2 pre-prepared Pie Crusts
1/2 cup Confectioner's Sugar
1/2 cup Skim Milk

Boil apples in two cups of water. While apples are cooking, roll pie crust into thin rectangular shapes and cut into 3x3 inch squares. Apples are ready if soft when stuck with fork. Drain apples in colander, then place in mixing bowl. Mash apples with potato masher. Add sugar and spices, mix well. Spoon 1-2 tablespoons of filling into the center of each square. Fold over into triangle shape, crimp edges of pastry with fork to seal. Place on cookie sheet sprayed with non-stick spray. Place in 350 degree oven for 20 minutes, or until crust is lightly browned. While turnovers are baking, make icing. Combine confectioner's sugar with skim milk. When turnovers are done, remove from oven, allow to cool for a few minutes, move onto serving dish and lightly pour sugar mixture over turnovers. Note: Applesauce can be made from any remaining filling by putting it into a food processor and pureeing it.

Number of Servings: 8
Nutritional Analysis Per Serving:
Calories: 185
Fat: 6 gm (28%)
Fiber: 1 gm
Cholesterol: -0-
Saturated Fat: 1 gm
Beta Carotene: 66 I.U.
Vitamin C: 4 mg

Blueberry Turnovers

2 cups cleaned, rinsed Blueberries

1/4 cup Sugar

1 pre-prepared Pie Crusts

1/2 cup Confectioner's Sugar

1/2 cup Skim Milk

Boil blueberries in two cups of water for 10 minutes. While blueberries are cooking, roll pie crust into thin rectangular shapes and cut into 3x3 inch squares. When blueberries are done, drain in colander, then place in mixing bowl. Mash with potato masher. Add sugar and mix well. Spoon 1 - 2 tablespoons of filling into the center of each square. Fold over into triangle shape, crimp edges of pastry with fork to seal. Place on cookie sheet sprayed with non-stick spray. Place in 350 degree oven for 20 minutes, or until crust is lightly browned. While turnovers are baking, make icing. Combine confectioner's sugar with skim milk. When turnovers are done, remove from oven, allow to cool for a few minutes, move onto serving dish and lightly pour sugar mixture over turnovers.

Number of Servings: 10
Nutritional Analysis Per Serving:
Calories: 135
Fat: 4 gm (31%)
Fiber: 1 gm
Cholesterol: -0-
Saturated Fat: 1 gm
Beta Carotene: 35 I.U.
Vitamin C: 4 mg

Bread Pudding

6 slices, toasted, cubed Whole Wheat Bread

1/2 cup Raisins

2 cups Skim Milk

2 Egg Whites

5 tablespoons Sugar

1 teaspoon Allspice

1 teaspoon Vanilla

Spread bread cubes evenly over bottom of casserole dish sprayed with non-stick spray. Sprinkle raisins over bread cubes. In a mixing bowl, combine skim milk, egg whites, sugar, allspice and vanilla. Use a fork to blend and whip well. Pour mixture over bread and raisins. Bake in 325 degree oven for 30 - 40 minutes. Remove from oven and test to see if done by inserting a knife. If it comes out clean, pudding is done; if not return to oven and check often. Cool before serving.

Number of Servings: 8
Nutritional Analysis Per Serving:
Calories: 132
Fat: less than 1 gm (6%)
Fiber: 1 gm
Cholesterol: 1 mg
Saturated Fat: less than 1 gm
Beta Carotene: 125 I.U.
Vitamin C: trace

Cantaloupe in Raspberry Sauce

1 ripe Cantaloupe

1 pint Raspberries

2 tablespoons Sugar

Cut cantaloupe into six equal pieces and scoop out seeds. In sauce pan, gently simmer raspberries in one cup of water. Stir raspberries frequently. When they are quite warm, add sugar and continue to simmer. Place pieces of cantaloupe on individual serving dishes and spoon raspberry sauce over cantaloupe.

Number of Servings: 4
Nutritional Analysis Per Serving:
Calories: 100
Fat: 1 gm (9%)
Fiber: 2 gm
Cholesterol: -0-
Saturated Fat: less than 1 gm
Beta Carotene: 2,000 I.U.
Vitamin C: 32 mg

Carrot Cake

2 cups all-purpose Flour

1 cup Sugar

1 teaspoon Baking Powder

1 teaspoon Baking Soda

1 teaspoon Allspice

2 tablespoons Safflower Oil

3 Egg Whites

3 cups finely shredded Carrots

1/2 cup Confectioner's Sugar

In a large mixing bowl combine flour, sugar, baking powder, baking soda and allspice. Mix well. Add oil, egg whites and carrots, using a mixer after each ingredient. Add combined dry ingredients a little at a time, mixing well after each addition. Turn into rectangular cake pan sprayed with non-stick spray. Bake in 325 degree oven for 45 minutes. Check with knife to see if done, if knife comes out clean it is done. If cake is not done, return to oven. Allow cake to cool when finished baking, then using a sifter, sprinkle confectioner's sugar over cake.

Number of Servings: 12
Nutritional Analysis Per Serving:
Calories: 185
Fat: 2 gm (12%)
Fiber: 1 gm
Cholesterol: -0-
Saturated Fat: less than 1 gm
Beta Carotene: 5,000 I.U.
Vitamin C: 2 mg

Fruit Pops

2 cups Strawberries or Blueberries

1 cup concentrated Apple Juice

1/2 cup cool Water

or

2 cups sectioned, seedless Oranges

1 cup concentrated Orange Juice

1/2 cup cool Water

In a blender combine fruit, juice and water. Puree until fine. Pour into freezer molds and freeze overnight.

Number of Servings: 4
Nutritional Analysis Per Serving, based on
Orange Fruit Pops:
Calories: 130
Fat: trace
Fiber: 0.5 gm
Cholesterol: -0-
Saturated Fat: less than 1 gm
Beta Carotene: 350 I.U.
Vitamin C: 66 mg

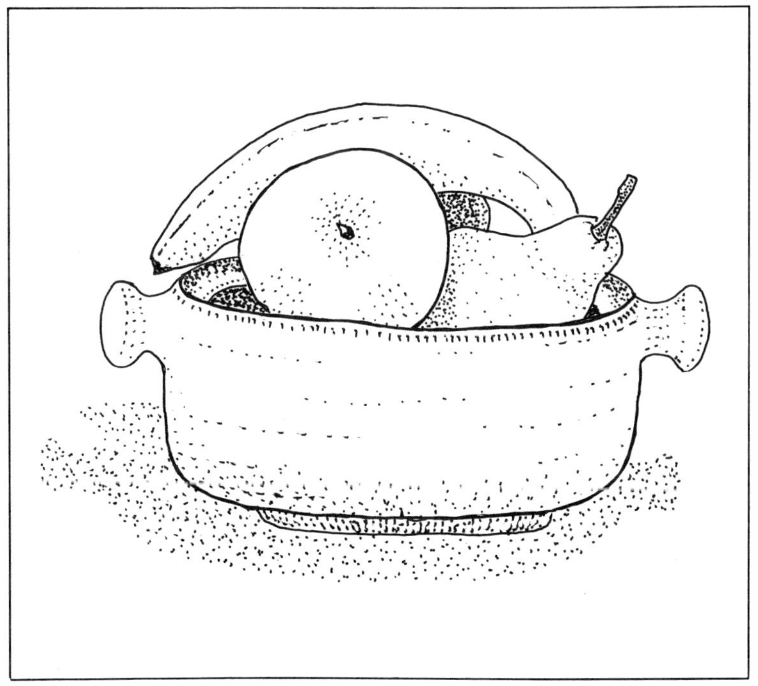

Fruit and Nut Salad

Fruit and Nut Salad

1 Cantaloupe

1 bunch, seedless Grapes

1 Honeydew Melon

2 peeled, thinly sliced Kiwi

6 peeled, sliced Oranges

2 pints Strawberries

2 pints Blueberries

1 tablespoon crushed Walnuts

Prepare as follows: half cantaloupe and honeydew melon, scoop out seeds and cut into small cubes or make balls. Wash and drain grapes, strawberries and blueberries through colander. Cut stems off of strawberries and slice in quarters. Combine all fruit into large mixing bowl. Careful to maintain as much of the fruit juice as possible while preparing fruit. Mix well. Mash just slightly with potato masher. Add nuts and stir well.

Number of Servings: 12
Nutritional Analysis Per Serving:
Calories: 144
Fat: 1 gm (7%)
Fiber: 3 gm
Cholesterol: -0-
Saturated Fat: less than 1 gm
Beta Carotene: 1,700 I.U.
Vitamin C: 110 mg

Minted Pears

1 can of halved Pears

1 teaspoon Mint Extract

1 bunch chopped Mint

Drain and arrange pears in serving dish. Combine mint extract with 1/2 cup cool water. Pour minted water completely over pears. Garnish with mint.

Number of Servings: 4
Nutritional Analysis Per Serving:
Calories: 65
Fat: -0-
Fiber: 1 gm
Cholesterol: -0-
Saturated Fat: -0-
Beta Carotene: 5 I.U.
Vitamin C: 5 mg

Pineapple Upside Down Cake and Sauce

1 cup Flour
1/2 cup Brown Sugar
2 teaspoons Baking Powder
1 teaspoon Cinnamon
2 Egg Whites
1 teaspoon Vanilla
1 8 oz. can of Pineapple Slices
1 8 oz. can of Crushed Pineapple

Drain juice from can of sliced pineapple and set aside. In large bowl combine flour, brown sugar, baking powder and cinnamon. Stir well. In a separate bowl, combine egg whites, vanilla and reserved pineapple juice. Using a whisk, mix well. Pour liquids into bowl of dry ingredients. Stir well. Open can of crushed pineapple and drain liquid. Stir crushed pineapple into batter. Arrange slices of pineapple in rectangular pan sprayed with non-stick spray. Pour batter over slices. Bake in 350 degree oven for 30 - 40 minutes or until cake has turned golden brown. Cool slightly after removing from oven. Invert onto serving platter.

Number of Servings: 12
Nutritional Analysis Per Serving:
Calories: 100
Fat: less than 1 gm (2%)
Fiber: less than 1 gm
Cholesterol: -0-
Saturated Fat: -0-
Beta Carotene: 12 I.U.
Vitamin C: 4 mg

Peach Cobbler

1 can of natural Peach Pie Filling

1 cup all-purpose Flour

1/2 cup Sugar

1 cup Old Fashioned Oats

1 tablespoon chopped Walnuts

1 tablespoon Cinnamon

2 tablespoons Margarine

1 Egg White

Dash of Salt

Pour peach filling into pan sprayed with non-stick spray. In a mixing bowl combine flour, sugar, oats, walnuts, cinnamon and a dash of salt. Cut margarine into mixture with a fork until it forms a crumb-like consistency. Add egg white and walnuts then mix well. Pour mixture over filling. Bake in 375 degree oven for 30 - 40 minutes or until topping becomes lightly brown.

Number of Servings: 12
Nutritional Analysis Per Serving:
Calories: 120
Fat: 1 gm (8%)
Fiber: less than 1 gm
Cholesterol: -0-
Saturated Fat: less than 1 gm
Beta Carotene: 185 I.U.
Vitamin C: 2 mg

Rice Pudding

2 cups cooked Brown Rice

2 cups Skim Milk

2 Egg Whites

3 tablespoons Honey

1 teaspoon Allspice

1 teaspoon Vanilla

1/2 cup Raisins

Combine all ingredients in large mixing bowl and mix well. Pour ingredients in casserole dish sprayed with non-stick spray, cover and bake at 325 degrees for 40 - 45 minutes.

Number of Servings: 6
Nutritional Analysis Per Serving:
Calories: 90
Fat: less than 1 gm (5%)
Fiber: 2 gm
Cholesterol: 1 mg
Saturated Fat: less than 1 gm
Beta Carotene: 170
Vitamin C: -0-

Cheesecake

1 cup Low-Fat Cottage Cheese

1 cup Skim Milk

1/2 cup Low-Fat Vanilla Yogurt

2 Egg Whites

3/4 cup Honey

1 teaspoon Vanilla

2 cups No-Oil Oatmeal Cookies

In a blender break up oatmeal cookies into fine pieces. Press into bottom of 9 - 10 inch pie pan. Break up cottage cheese. Add milk and vanilla yogurt, mix until smooth. Add egg whites one at a time. Add honey and vanilla, mix well. Pour into prepared pie shell. Cover and bake in 325 degree oven for 1 hour or until lightly brown and firm.

Number of Servings: 12
Nutritional Analysis Per Serving:
Calories: 140
Fat: less than 1 gm (2%)
Fiber: 2 gm
Cholesterol: 2 mg
Saturated Fat: less than 1 gm
Beta Carotene: 55 I.U.
Vitamin C: -0-

Strawberry Short Cake

1 package of 6 No-Fat Dessert Shells

1 pint Strawberries

1 tablespoon Sugar

1 pint Non-Fat Frozen Vanilla Yogurt

Wash and drain strawberries in colander. Remove stem from each strawberry and cut into quarters. Set several quarters aside for garnish later on. Using a potato masher, mash the remaining strawberries well, add sugar and stir well. Spoon strawberry mixture onto individual dessert shells. Spoon frozen yogurt on top of strawberries. Garnish with remaining strawberry quarters.

Number of Servings: 6
Nutritional Analysis Per Serving:
Calories: 190
Fat: less than 1 gm (2%)
Fiber: less than 1 gm
Cholesterol: 1 mg
Saturated Fat: less than 1 gm
Beta Carotene: 20 I.U.
Vitamin C: 17 mg

Lemon Sorbet

2 cups Non-Fat Vanilla Yogurt

3/4 cup concentrated Lemon Juice

1 tablespoon Yellow Food Coloring

Combine all above ingredients in metal mixing bowl. Using mixer, whip until creamy. Cover and put bowl in freezer for 15 minutes. Remove from freezer and whip briefly with mixer. Continue to freeze and mix until sorbet becomes stiff and creamy.

Number of Servings: 4
Nutritional Analysis Per Serving:
Calories: 75
Fat: trace
Fiber: -0-
Cholesterol: 2 mg
Saturated Fat: less than 1 gm
Beta Carotene: 20 I.U.
Vitamin C: 56 mg

Strawberry Sorbet

3 cups Non-Fat Vanilla Yogurt

1 pint Strawberries

2 tablespoons Sugar

Wash and drain strawberries in colander. Remove stem from each strawberry. Place strawberries in blender with sugar and puree until smooth. Put strawberries and yogurt in metal mixing bowl. Using a mixer, whip until creamy. Cover and put bowl in freezer for 15 minutes. Remove from freezer and whip briefly with mixer. Continue to freeze and mix until sorbet becomes stiff and creamy.

Number of Servings: 6
Nutritional Analysis Per Serving:
Calories: 92
Fat: less than 1 gm (3%)
Fiber: less than 1 gm
Cholesterol: 2 mg
Saturated Fat: less than 1 gm
Beta Carotene: 23 I.U.
Vitamin C: 18 mg

Raspberry Sorbet

3 cups Non-Fat Vanilla Yogurt

1 pint Raspberries

2 tablespoons Sugar

Wash and drain raspberries in colander. Place raspberries in blender with sugar and puree until smooth. Put raspberries and yogurt in metal mixing bowl. Using a mixer, whip until creamy. Cover and put bowl in freezer for 15 minutes. Remove from freezer and whip briefly with mixer. Continue to freeze and mix until sorbet becomes stiff and creamy.

Number of Servings: 6
Nutritional Analysis Per Serving:
Calories: 97
Fat: less than 1 gm (3%)
Fiber: 1 gm
Cholesterol: 2 mg
Saturated Fat: less than 1 gm
Beta Carotene: 63 I.U.
Vitamin C: 7 mg

Banana Bread

4 very ripe, mashed Bananas

2 cups all-purpose Flour

1 teaspoon Baking Powder

1/2 teaspoon Baking Soda

1/2 cup Sugar

1 teaspoon Vanilla

2 Egg Whites

In a large bowl, stir together flour, baking powder, and baking soda. In a separate bowl, with a mixer blend together sugar, vanilla and egg whites. Add bananas to sugar mixture. When thoroughly mixed, begin to add small amounts of the flour mixture to banana mixture. Continue until completely blended. Pour batter into loaf pan sprayed with non-stick spray. Bake in 350 degree oven for 45 - 50 minutes or until done. Test by sticking knife into center of loaf, if it comes out clean it is done. If top starts to brown a little too quickly, cover loosely with tin foil and continue to bake.

Number of Servings: 12
Nutritional Analysis Per Serving:
Calories: 150
Fat: less than 1 gm (3%)
Fiber: less than 1 gm
Cholesterol: -0-
Saturated Fat: less than 1 gm
Beta Carotene: 30 I.U.
Vitamin C: 3 mg

Bran Muffins

1 cup Bran Cereal

1 cup all-purpose Flour

2 teaspoons Baking Powder

2 tablespoons Sugar

1 cup Skim Milk

1 tablespoon Safflower Oil

1 Egg White

In a large bowl, stir together flour, baking powder and sugar. In a separate bowl, mix together milk, oil and egg white. Add bran cereal to milk mixture and allow to set for 2 minutes then stir well. Add a small amount of flour mixture to bran mixture, blend well with mixer. Continue to combine until both mixtures are completely blended. Pour batter into muffin pans sprayed with non-stick spray. Bake in 350 degree oven for 20 - 25 minutes or until done. Test by sticking knife into center of a muffin, if it comes out clean it is done. If top starts to brown a little too quickly, cover loosely with tin foil and continue to bake.

Number of Servings: 12
Nutritional Analysis Per Serving:
Calories: 110
Fat: 2 gm (15%)
Fiber: 6 gm
Cholesterol: -0-
Saturated Fat: -0-
Beta Carotene: 1,000 I.U.
Vitamin C: -0-

Corn Bread

1 cup all-purpose Flour
1 cup Yellow Corn Meal
2 teaspoons Baking Powder
1 teaspoon Cinnamon
2 tablespoons Sugar
1 cup Skim Milk
1 tablespoon Safflower Oil
1 Egg White
Dash of Salt

In a large bowl, stir together flour, baking powder, cinnamon, sugar and salt. In a separate bowl, mix together milk, oil and egg white. Add corn meal to milk mixture and allow to set for 2 minutes then stir well. Add a small amount of flour mixture to corn meal mixture, blend well with mixer. Continue to combine until both mixtures are completely blended. Pour batter into shallow pan sprayed with non-stick spray. Bake in 400 degree oven for 20 - 25 minutes or until done. Test by sticking knife into center of bread, if it comes out clean it is done. If top starts to brown a little too quickly, cover loosely with tin foil and continue to bake.

Number of Servings: 12
Nutritional Analysis Per Serving:
Calories: 100
Fat: 2 gm (15%)
Fiber: 1 gm
Cholesterol: -0-
Saturated Fat: -0-
Beta Carotene: 100 I.U.
Vitamin C: trace

Dessert Crepes

1 cup all-purpose Flour

1 1/2 cups Skim Milk

2 Egg Whites

1 tablespoon Safflower Oil

2 tablespoons Sugar

Dash of Salt

Combine all of the above ingredients in a large mixing bowl. Mix with mixer until completely blended and smooth. Spray 6 inch skillet with non-stick spray. Heat pan slightly. Remove from heat. Spoon in 2 tablespoons of batter. Tilt skillet to spread batter until it covers bottom of pan evenly. Return pan to heat. Brown crepe on only one side. To remove crepe, invert pan onto plate covered with a paper towel. To make more crepes, repeat process making sure that pan maintains non-stick surface.

Number of Servings: 6
Nutritional Analysis Per Serving:
Calories: 135
Fat: 3 gm (16%)
Fiber: -0-
Cholesterol: 1 mg
Saturated Fat: less than 1 gm
Beta Carotene: 125 I.U.
Vitamin C: trace

French Baguettes

3 cups all-purpose Flour

1 package of Active Dry Yeast

1 1/2 teaspoons Salt

Put 1 cup warm water in a large mixing bowl and sprinkle yeast over water. Allow to set for 5 minutes or until water starts to look bubbly. Using a fork whisk 1 1/12 cup of flour and 3/4 teaspoon salt into water. Soak dish towel in warm water, wring out water, cover bowl with towel, set in warm place and allow to rise for several hours. Knead in remaining salt and as much of the remaining flour as possible into the dough. Pour leftover flour onto work surface and knead for 15 minutes or until dough is smooth, soft and elastic. Place dough in bowl sprayed with non-stick spray, cover with towel, set in a warm place and allow to rise until double in size. Punch down dough and allow to set for 5 - 10 minutes. Cut dough in half. Flatten dough with hands. Fold in half. Fold in half again in the other direction. And fold in half again in first direction. Roll with hands on work surface until dough becomes approximately 12 inches long and cylindrical in shape. Place seam-side down on cookie sheet sprayed with non-stick spray. Cover and allow to rise for 30 minutes. Preheat oven to 450 degrees. Cut four slanted gashes with a very sharp knife in the top of each loaf.

Bake for 15 minutes. Turn heat down in oven and continue to bake in 350 degree oven for 20 minutes or until bread is golden brown. Cool for several minutes before attempting to cut. For extra crustiness baste with salt water every 5 minutes while baking.

Number of Servings: 12
Nutritional Analysis Per Serving:
Calories: 100
Fat: less than 1 gm (2%)
Fiber: 1 gm
Cholesterol: -0-
Saturated Fat: less than 1 gm
Beta Carotene: trace
Vitamin C: -0-

Pumpkin Bread

2 cups all-purpose Flour
2 teaspoons Baking Powder
1/4 teaspoon Baking Soda
1/2 teaspoon Cinnamon
1 teaspoon Allspice
1/2 cup Brown Sugar
1/4 cup Skim Milk
1/4 cup Safflower Oil
2 Egg Whites
1 cup of canned Pumpkin

In a large mixing bowl combine flour, baking powder, baking soda, cinnamon and allspice. Set aside. In a separate bowl combine brown sugar, milk, oil and egg whites. Using a mixer blend until smooth. Add pumpkin and mix until well combined. Add a small amount of the flour mixture to the pumpkin mixture and mix well. Continue this process until all ingredients are completely blended. Pour batter into loaf pan sprayed with non-stick spray. Bake in 350 degree oven for 60 minutes or until done. Test by sticking knife into center of bread, if it comes out clean it is done. If top starts to brown a little too quickly, cover loosely with tin foil and continue to bake.

Number of Servings: 10
Nutritional Analysis Per Serving:
Calories: 187
Fat: 6 gm (29%)
Fiber: 1.5 gm
Cholesterol: trace
Saturated Fat: 0.6 gm
Beta Carotene: 5,417 I.U.
Vitamin C: 1.0 mg

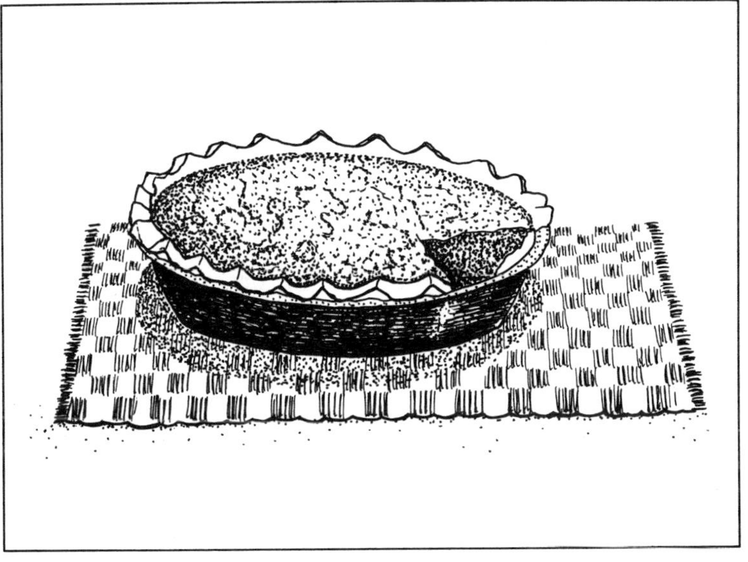

Pumpkin Pie

Pumpkin Pie

1 16 oz. can of Pumpkin

1 5 oz. can of Evaporated Skim Milk

1/2 cup Skim Milk

2 Egg Whites

1 teaspoon Cinnamon

1/2 teaspoon Nutmeg

1 teaspoon Allspice

1 teaspoon Vanilla

2 cups No-Oil Oatmeal Cookies

Combine all above ingredients, except pumpkin, in one bowl and whip with fork. Add pumpkin and blend with mixer until smooth and creamy. To prepare pie crust, break up oatmeal cookies into fine pieces in blender. Pour crumbs into 9 - 10 inch pie pan and press into pan. Pour filling into crust. Cover pie with foil and bake in 450 degree oven for 10 minutes. Uncover pie and continue to bake in 350 degree oven for 20 - 30 minutes or until done. Pie is done when knife inserted in center comes out clean. Cool pie for several minutes before serving.

Number of Servings: 6
Nutritional Analysis Per Serving:
Calories: 79
Fat: 1 gm (11%)
Fiber: 4 gm
Cholesterol: 1 mg
Saturated Fat: trace
Beta Carotene: 18,138 I.U.
Vitamin C: 5 mg

Beverages

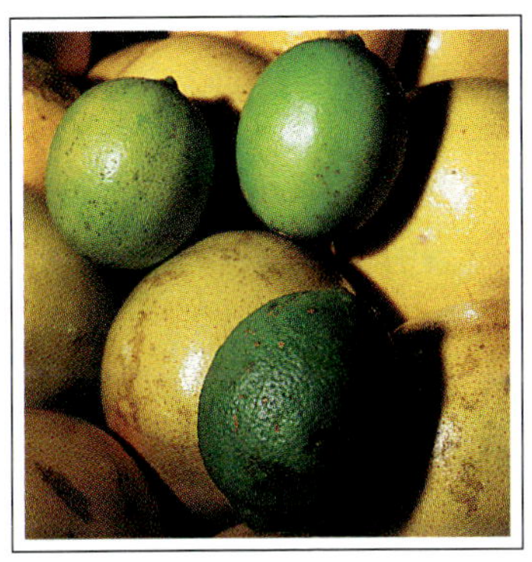

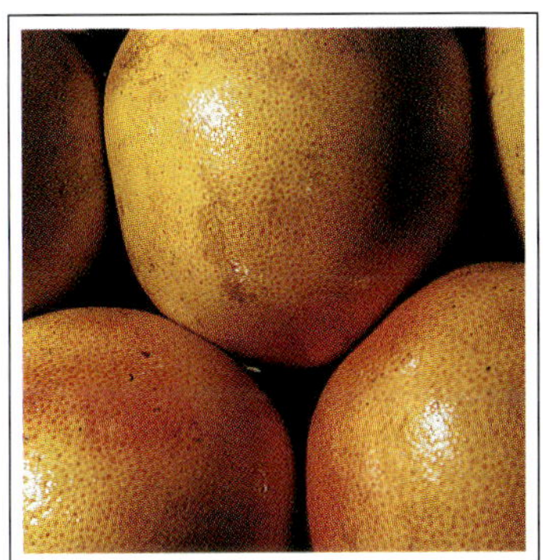

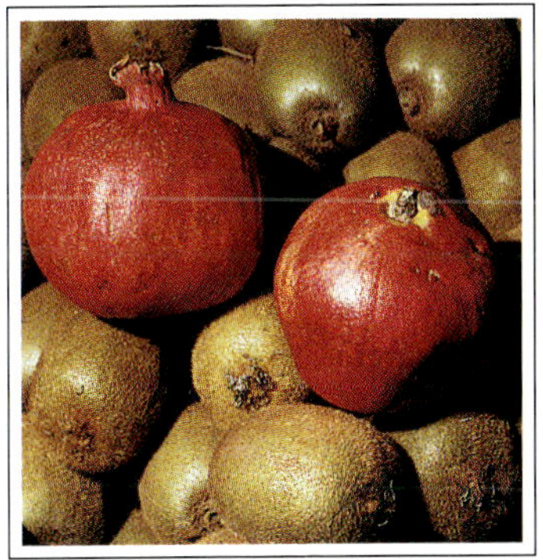

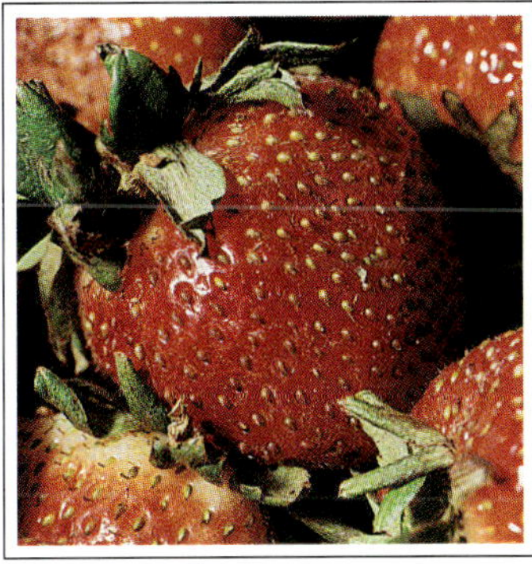

Fruit Drinks

Orange-Cranberry

1 cup Orange Juice

1 cup Cranberry Juice

or

Pineapple-Orange-Banana

1 cup Pineapple/Orange Juice

1 Banana

or

Strawberry-Banana

1 cup frozen Strawberries

1 Banana

or

Blueberry-Apple

1 cup frozen Blueberries

1 cup Apple Juice

and

1/2 cup Non-Fat Vanilla Yogurt

5 Ice Cubes

(Continued on next page)

Combine any of the above suggested combinations with yogurt and ice cubes in a blender. Blend until frothy.

Number of Servings: 6
Nutritional Analysis Per Serving,
based on Pineapple-Orange-Banana Fruit Drink:
Calories: 50
Fat: less than 1 gm (3%)
Fiber: -0-
Cholesterol: -0-
Saturated Fat: -0-
Beta Carotene: 60 I.U.
Vitamin C: 14 mg

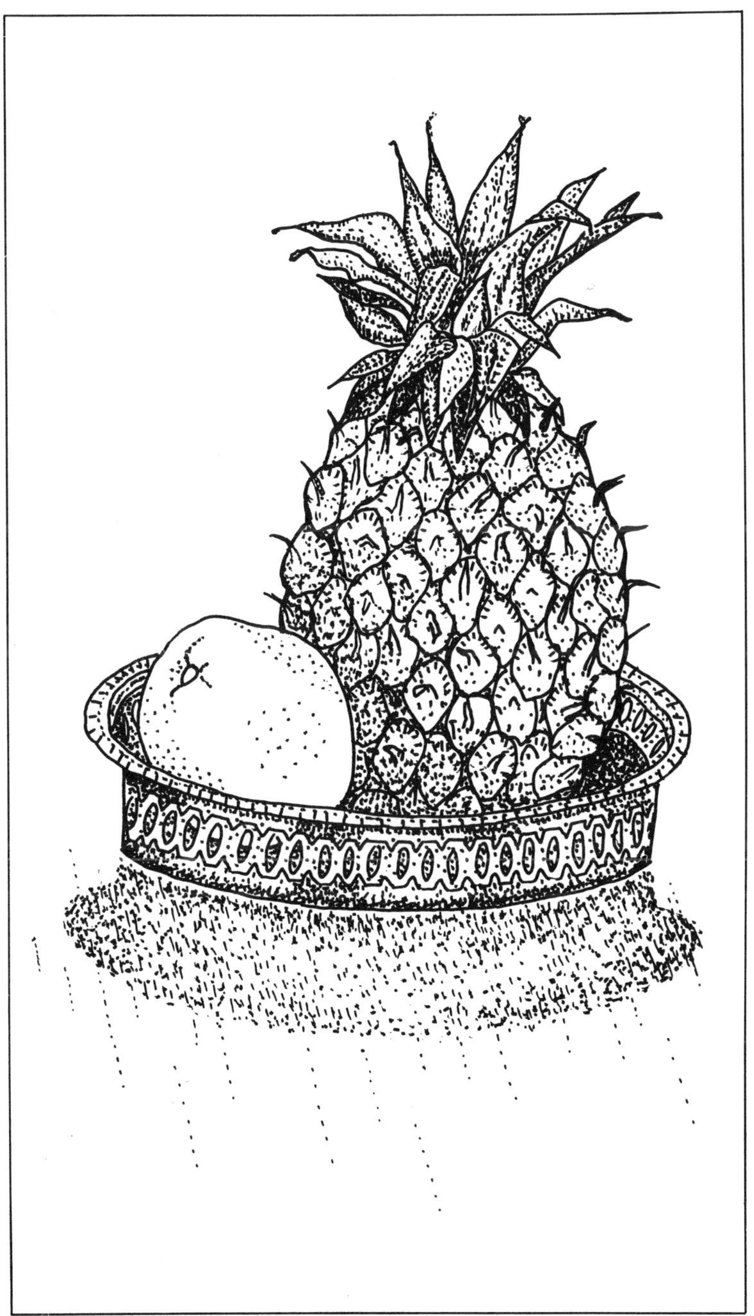

Fruit Drinks

Orange Fiz

1 cup Orange Juice

1 cup No-Cal Orange Soda

1/2 cup Non-Fat Dry Milk

4 Ice Cubes

Combine all above ingredients in blender until frothy.

Number of Servings: 6
Nutritional Analysis Per Serving:
Calories: 90
Fat: less than 1 gm (2%)
Fiber: -0-
Cholesterol: 3 mg
Saturated Fat: less than 1 gm
Beta Carotene: 443 I.U.
Vitamin C: 20 mg

Sangría (no alcohol)

1 thinly sliced Orange

1 thinly sliced Lemon

1 cup halved Grapes

3 tablespoons Lemon Juice

1 small can of frozen Orange Juice

1 small can of frozen Cranberry Juice

1 quart chilled Carbonated Water

5 pieces of Ice

Combine all juices and stir well. Just before serving add carbonated water, fruit and ice. Stir gently.

Number of Servings: 8
Nutritional Analysis Per Serving:
Calories: 50
Fat: -0-
Fiber: -0-
Cholesterol: -0-
Saturated Fat: -0-
Beta Carotene: 140 I.U.
Vitamin C: 50 mg

About The Cancer Research Foundation of America

The Cancer Research Foundation of America was founded in 1985 by a group of individuals concerned that, although the previous decade had yielded tremendous advances in the war against cancer, the results were not being reported to the American public in a meaningful way. The general perception was that billions of dollars had been spent on cancer research, but very little progress had been made. We felt this perception needed changing.

We also believed there was much information now known about cancer prevention which was not reaching the average American - such as the fact that as much as 70% of cancer is now considered to be preventable. We felt this information could and should be distributed to help teach everyone how to lower their risk of getting cancer. Many Americans do not know that diet is strongly linked to cancer; in fact, the National Cancer Institute estimates that about 35% of all cancer cases are diet related.

In 1971 the president of the United States officially declared War on Cancer. The goal of this campaign is to reduce cancer deaths by half before the year 2000. We believe that the best way to reach this goal is by helping prevent cancer from occurring in the first place. Thus CRFA established its highest priority: the prevention of cancer. Our programs are focused on cancer prevention at all levels including:

- **basic research on dietary links to cancer**
- **prevention of recurrence of cancer through innovative new treatments and dietary changes**

- **prevention of advanced stage cancer through early detection**
- **education of the public on cancer risk and how each individual can reduce this risk**

Because such great progress has been made in treating childhood cancers, we believe it to be critically important to continue funding research in this field. What better legacy would we leave future generations than to help eradicate cancer in children and teach them to prevent it as adults? Thus we developed our dual commitment to cancer prevention and cancer in children.

CRFA has awarded research grants to many of the leading cancer centers and universities in the United States, but we are also committed to funding small, grass-roots organizations that sometimes "fall through the cracks" when seeking federal grants. We seek out organizations of people helping people prevent and learn about cancer. We look for programs that will aim for a dollar's worth of effort for every dollar we award.

CRFA is committed to efficiency - both in the projects we fund and in our own organization. We believe that any gift to CRFA is a public trust and should be used as wisely and efficiently as possible. We are grateful for your support, and we pledge to use your gifts to fight cancer, not to operate our foundation.

1990 was another year of tremendous growth and accomplishment for the Cancer Research Foundation of America (CRFA). There has been a significant increase in the public's awareness of and support for the foundation, judged by the volume of mail received at our headquarters. At the end of the year, CRFA members numbered nearly four hundred thousand.

During 1989, CRFA recorded a significant achievement: selection for participation in the Combined Federal

Campaign the first year we were eligible. This means that federal workers are now given the opportunity to support CRFA through regular payroll deductions. We believe this will be a valuable source of support for our programs for years to come.

Additionally, CRFA continued to meet all standards for wise giving of the major national organizations that monitor charitable fund raising activity.

During 1990, researchers at leading cancer centers and other medical institutions were contacted by CRFA and invited to submit grant proposals. The medical and scientific communities have also become increasingly aware of CRFA, and the number of grant proposals received has continued to rise. Our Medical Advisory Board has helped bring the Foundation to the attention of their colleagues and has reviewed basic research proposals, fellowship applications, and educational projects of the highest quality.

The foundation has continued its commitment to seek out worthy organizations which have found it difficult to obtain funds from traditional sources. We are proud of this involvement with "grass-roots" groups, many of which are using scarce funds even more efficiently and productively than some of the better known institutions. Personal contact with all CRFA grant recipients helps us ensure that funds for each project will be used wisely.

CRFA's achievements are many. Grants to scientists at major universities and cancer centers particularly emphasized research aimed at preventing the three major cancer killers: cancer of the colon, lung, and breast. Together, these three account for nearly half the cancer deaths in men and women nationally.

CRFA remains committed to operating an efficient organization which will make more of its funds available for the research and educational programs approved by our Board of Directors. In 1990 administrative expenses represented just over 1% of the total funds raised by CRFA during the year.

The foundation seeks no governmental funding, to the contrary, several of its grants represented supplemental funding to that received from the federal government. The National Cancer Institute received a grant from the CRFA, so that yet another promising young scientist could pursue a research career without the constant concern about cutbacks in federal funding.

We have continued our nationwide project entitled "Your Cancer Risk," an educational program designed to alert individuals about cancer risk and how it can be reduced. We estimate that our materials reached more than ten million Americans in 1989. We believe that Americans need to be continually reminded that as much as 70% of all cancer is preventable -- yet less than one-third of 1% of the medical care budget in the United States goes toward prevention.

The Board of Directors is particularly proud of our CRFA Research Fellowship Program, which we believe will enable some of the brightest young minds to participate in cancer research rather than leave the laboratory and pursue a career elsewhere, forced out by a lack of funding. Fellowship funding was continued at the University of California at Los Angeles, the George Washington University School of Medicine, Cornell University, the Wistar Institute, and the Veterans Administration Medical Center in Washington, DC. Many of these awards have been renewed for a second year, providing the continuity in research programs that is often lacking when a one-year fellow moves on.

New fellowships were awarded to researchers at the National Cancer Institute, Georgetown University's Vincent T. Lombardi Cancer Research Center, the American Health Foundation and the University of Texas

Anderson Foundation Cancer Center. These new fellowships and nearly all the renewals were in the areas of colon, lung, and breast cancer.

Our newsletter *The CRFA Monitor* is published quarterly; each issue brings up-to-date information about progress in cancer research to at least one million individuals. It also contains practical information about reducing cancer risk, including material on diet and nutrition and their link to cancer prevention. *The Monitor* informs our generous supporters about how their gifts are being used, and features articles about specific CRFA grant recipients. In addition over 10,000 copies of Dr. Oliver Alabaster's ground breaking book *The Power of Prevention* have been distributed through *The Monitor*. This book offers readers concise and enlightening information on how they can reduce cancer risk for themselves, friends and family.

Our continued commitment to funding worthy "grass-roots" organizations included the grants to ANRF and STAT as well as to the Wisconsin Cancer Pain Initiative. Cancer pain and its prevention were the subject of a CRFA grant to the Medical College of Wisconsin to educate physicians on the often overlooked subject. Another project that reaches individuals at the grass-roots level is the training of public health nurses at the University of West Virginia Mary Babb Randolph Cancer Center. These nurses learned to perform pap smears and teach breast self-examination to women in rural areas with little or no access to medical care.

Childhood cancer continues to be a priority for CRFA, demonstrated by grants to the pediatric branch of the National Cancer Institute for work in Burkitt's lymphoma, to the Rainbow Babies and Childrens Hospital of Case Western Reserve University for studies on childhood leukemia, and to Childrens' Hospice International for continuation of its highly successful toll-free hotline, which is making a real difference in the care of terminally ill young people.

Our efforts to help prevent lung cancer also includes support for programs aimed at keeping adolescents from smoking - or to help them quit if they have already begun to smoke. These grants include continued support for the "Teens as Teachers" program developed by the American Non-Smokers' Rights Foundation (ANRF), educational programs conducted by two counties in New Jersey, and efforts of the group Stop Teenage Addiction to Tobacco (STAT).

Having begun the decade with such an excellent response from our members, the CRFA can confidently look forward to even greater achievement in waging the battle against cancer in America.

For more information about the Cancer Research Foundation of America, its newsletter the *Monitor*, other publications, programs, or to make a donation, contact:

The Cancer Research Foundation of America

700 Princess Street, Suite 5

Alexandria, Virginia 22314

(703) 836-4412

Index

S

T

V

W

Y